365 WAYS TO
BOOST YOUR
BRAIN POWER

365 WAYS TO BOOST YOUR BRAIN POWER

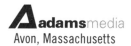

Tips. Exercises. Advice.

Carolyn Dean, M.D., Valentine Dmitriev, Ph.D., and Donna Raskin

▲adamsmedia
Avon, Massachusetts

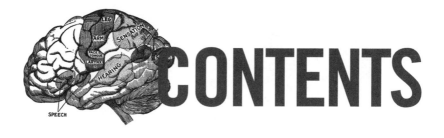

CONTENTS

V

CHAPTER 3: FEED YOUR BRAIN—BASICS 23

CHAPTER 5: FEED YOUR BRAIN—SUPERFOODS 67

CHAPTER 6: SUPPLEMENT YOUR BRAIN WITH HERBS 81

CHAPTER 7: NOURISH YOUR BRAIN WITH MINERALS 95

CHAPTER 8: **REPLENISH YOUR BRAIN WITH VITAMINS** 111

CHAPTER 14: REJUVENATE YOUR BRAIN 173

CHAPTER 15: STIMULATE YOUR BRAIN 179

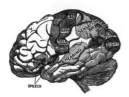

QUIZ

How well are you treating your brain?

How much do you know about your own brain and what it requires to function well? Do you eat with your brain in mind? Do you take protective measures to keep your mind nimble well into old age? Do you pamper or do you abuse your brain? Take the following quiz to find out where you stand with your brain. Choose the answer that's closest to true for you.

1. HOW OFTEN DO YOU EXERCISE?

a. At least six days a week, lifting weights two days and brisk walking at least three miles the other four.

b. Once or twice a week I take a long walk.

c. I rarely exercise.

2. DO YOU EAT A VARIETY OF FRUITS AND VEGETABLES?

a. I love them and eat a wide variety of both fruits and vegetables every day.

b. I eat my favorites—carrots, green beans, squash, tomatoes, oranges, and bananas.

c. I don't really like vegetables, unless you consider potatoes a vegetable.

3. HOW OFTEN DO YOU EAT FISH?

a. I eat wild salmon once a week, and at least one other fresh fish a week.
b. I eat fish occasionally, but prefer meat or chicken.
c. I don't like fish and never eat it, unless you count the occasional fish sandwich at McDonald's.

4. HOW OFTEN AND WHAT DO YOU DRINK?

a. I typically have one glass of red wine with dinner one or two nights a week.
b. I like two glasses of wine with dinner, followed by an aperitif occasionally.
c. I mostly binge drink hard liquor and beer on the weekends.

5. DO YOU KNOW YOUR HDL AND LDL NUMBERS?

a. Yes, I check them regularly and work to raise my HDL and lower my LDL by monitoring my diet and exercising often.
b. I had them checked five years ago, but I have no idea what they are now.
c. What are HDL and LDL?

6. DO YOU HAVE A METHOD FOR DEALING WITH STRESS?

a. I take yoga classes twice a week; meditate for 15 minutes each day; keep a journal; and take concrete measures to reduce stress.
b. Not really, I typically crash on the sofa when I get home with a glass of wine until I feel relaxed.
c. I have a very demanding job (that I hate) and three kids so stress is constant and time for myself nonexistent.

7. HOW OFTEN DO YOU SOCIALIZE?

a. I belong to a book club that meets once a week, attend church regularly, volunteer once a week, and invite friends and new acquaintances over for dinner often.
b. I hang out with the same group of friends once a week or so.
c. I don't have the time or energy to socialize.

8. HOW OFTEN DO YOU HAVE SEX?

a. At least three times a week.
b. Two to four times a month.
c. I'm not in a relationship so very rarely.

9. WHEN WAS THE LAST TIME YOU LEARNED SOMETHING NEW OR CHALLENGING?

a. I'm always trying something new. Right now I'm taking piano and French lessons, plus a class in sculpture just for fun.
b. When I was in college ten years ago.
c. Why learn anything new? I like to stay with the tried and true.

10. WHEN IS THE LAST TIME YOU READ A BOOK?

a. I read constantly and am particularly fond of historical or literary fiction and Shakespearean sonnets.
b. I read magazines and popular novels at the beach in the summer.
c. I rarely read. Why read when you can watch TV?

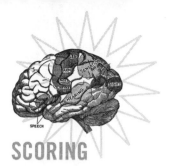

SCORING

For every **a** answer, give yourself 2 points.
For every **b** answer, give yourself 1 point.
For every **c** answer, give yourself 0 points.

15–20 points: You're doing a lot of things right, and your brain loves you for it . . . but there's always room for improvement.

9–14 points: You're lagging behind but can turn things around with a little effort. Hopefully you'll find a lot of motivation in the forthcoming pages.

0–8 points: Your brain is crying out for attention. You need to take this book to heart before your brain goes to seed.

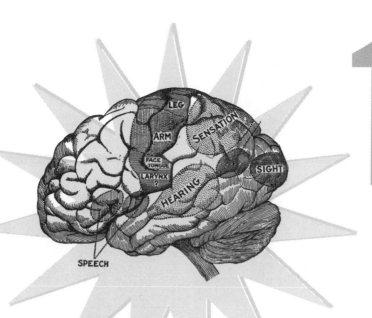

KNOW
YOUR
BRAIN

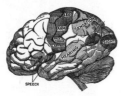

KNOW YOUR BRAIN

The brain is a supercomputer, the likes of which will probably never be duplicated by technology.

1. UNDERSTAND THE IMPORTANCE OF YOUR BRAIN

If you're going to keep your brain functioning well throughout your life, it's important that you know how it works. Virtually every aspect of your existence—physical, mental, and emotional—is governed by the three-pound mass of pinkish-gray tissue safely encased within your skull. Your brain is an extremely complex and miraculous organ that labors night and day to keep your alive, vital, and brilliant. Knowing the basics about how your brain works should inspire you to tend to its care and feeding. There is much to be said for visualization; hopefully, it will acquaint you with your brain—the most precious computer you'll ever own—and give you impetus to keep it hard-wired and functioning at its maximum capacity.

2. ENVISION YOUR BRAIN

Put your two palms together and then make your hands into fists. If you look down at your thumbs, you can envision the actual size of your brain. Your curled up fingers even look a bit like the incredible convolutions in the brain. Its 100 billion nerve cells weigh about three pounds in total and connect with each other along 100 trillion different pathways. The 100 billion nerve cells in the brain look like bizarre amoeba on hallucinogenic drugs. They have a central body where metabolism takes place, and they have several incredibly long, stretched-out arms, or axons, that conduct electrical signals. At the tips of the axons is where signals jump from one nerve cell to another. That junction is called a synapse; there are 100 trillion synapses in the brain.

3. HONOR YOUR BRAIN

The brain is a supercomputer, the likes of which will probably never be duplicated by technology. Just think of all the functions it's involved in: myriad memories, a wide range of moods, sensory perceptions (taste, touch, smell), all muscle movements, breathing, blood circulation, digestion, pressure, pain, swallowing, arousal, abstract thinking, identity, and more. And yes, we take it for granted—that is, until we find we are losing our grasp on it.

4. UNDERSTAND HOW YOUR BRAIN WORKS

Nerve cells in the brain communicate with one another and pass messages along the chain of command to keep the body functioning. Each of the 100 billion nerve cells has several axons or long arms attached. From those axons come multiple smaller arms called dendrites. A nerve cell, like all other cells, has a nucleus in the cell body that controls all the metabolic functions of the cell. The axon, which is the width of a hair, carries messages from one nerve cell to the next. Dendrites also receive messages from axons. Surrounding each nerve cell are neuroglial cells that provide nutrients, support, and protection. The nerve cells send and receive electrical messages. An electrical charge builds up in the nerve cell and then at a certain critical point it travels down to the end of its axon. At the tip of the axon a chemical messenger is released by the electrical stimulation.

Chemical messengers are called neurotransmitters. Their job is to travel the short distance from the tip of the axon to bind to receptor sites on dendrites or nerve cell bodies. The junction is called a synapse, and the average nerve cell has about 15,000 synapses. Now, aren't you impressed? Give your brain its due—it's a miraculous organ.

5. RESPECT YOUR ELDERS

Cells in the lining of our mouth and intestines live for only a few days; red blood cells live an average of three months. But nerve cells, which arise when we are in our mother's womb, are very long-lived. In fact, they can live 100 years or longer. We used to think that once nerve cells died they weren't replaced, but recent studies show that new nerve cells can arise in a few regions of the brain, even in older brains. This puts a whole new emphasis on how we can best support and stimulate the production of new nerve cells. Even so, as with anything that is going to be around for a long time, we must make sure to take good care of our nerve cells. The brain and body do their jobs by ensuring an ongoing process of cellular detoxification and repair. So, cherish those brain cells and keep them awake and alive.

6. EMBRACE THE WHOLE PACKAGE

The brain is divided into the right cerebral hemisphere and the left cerebral hemisphere and comprises 85 percent of your brain's weight. The connection between the cerebral hemispheres is called the corpus callosum and resembles a major telephone switching station crowded with bundles of nerve connections. The outer layer of the cerebral hemispheres is called the cerebral cortex and has an average thickness of ⅛ of an inch. It scans incoming sensations, and originates movement and thinking. The cerebellum (10 percent of the total brain volume) sits at the base of the brain and controls balance and coordination. The brain stem (5 percent) sits below the cerebellum where it relays messages from the brain to the spinal cord. It's crucial for automatic functions in the body such as breathing, heart rate, blood pressure, and sleep. The limbic system controls instinct, emotions, and the sense of smell. The thalamus receives information from the limbic system and transmits it to the cerebral cortex. The hippocampus converts short-term memories into long-term memories for storage. Alzheimer's plaques, for example, begin in the cortex near the hippocampus and then enter the hippocampus. Memory loss is often the first sign of Alzheimer's. ✳

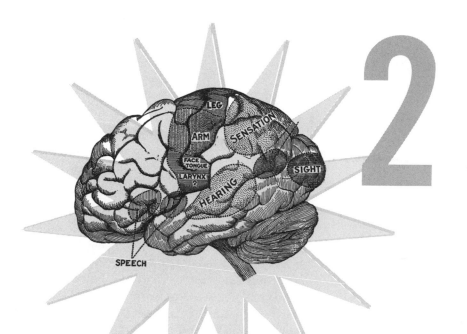

PROTECT YOUR BRAIN

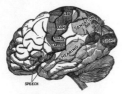

PROTECT YOUR BRAIN

"Mind, body, and spirit are inseparable."

7. TAKE RESPONSIBILITY

Given instantaneous relief of what ailed them, people gradually gave up responsibility for their own health. The advantage of modern pharmacopoeia was that people could abdicate responsibility for how they lived their lives, for what they ate, and how much; for what they imbibed, and how much; for how they worked, and how much; for the games they played and so forth. Unhealthy habits could be enjoyed, and their deleterious results could always be magically removed by a little colored pill. No need to develop *awareness* of one's own complexity—body, mind, emotions, and spirits, and how they interact. Someone else was trained to "know" what to do when you got into any kind of trouble. That the treatments didn't work—neither the medical nor the psychological— was easily ignored. It is up to you to know what's good for your brain and what isn't good for your brain.

8. THINK HOLISTICALLY

By this point in time we all know that our emotional, mental, and physical selves are intertwined and interlinked. We have ample evidence to prove that our psychological

8

health affects our physical health, and vice versa. It's vital to your overall health and your brain's health to think holistically—to view yourself as a whole being, not a collection of parts. In the 1970s when Buddhist ideas seeped into western culture one essential message was: "I am not my liver, my spleen, my blood, nor my brain. I am all of me." It sounded new and often revolutionary at the time, but science soon joined the chorus. You are not the sum of all your parts; you are the sum of all parts operating in tandem. Mind, body, and spirit are inseparable, and illness in one often produces illness in the others. Think holistically and your overall health, as well as your brain's health, will improve.

9. LOSE 10 PERCENT OF YOUR EXCESS BODY WEIGHT

Losing just 5 to 10 percent of excess body weight can help to reduce your risk for health problems related to your weight. It lowers blood pressure, total cholesterol, LDL cholesterol (bad cholesterol), triglyceride levels, and blood sugar. Lifestyle change is the healthiest and most permanent method of losing weight and decreasing the risk for serious health problems. Combining a healthy diet with increased physical activity and behavior modification is the most successful strategy for healthy weight loss and weight maintenance.

10. MINIMIZE ALCOHOL CONSUMPTION

Watch out for alcohol and other mind-numbing drugs. Most experts agree that a drink a day isn't health-threatening, but abuse of alcohol or recreational drugs can diminish your ability to absorb stimuli from the world around you and result in a limited ability to form new memories. Brain scans of alcoholics tend to show low activity in the cerebellum, the brain's major coordination center. Alcohol should be consumed in moderation—preferably one drink every few days and a maximum of one or two glasses a day. Because it is considered a neurotoxin, more than two glasses of alcohol a day can adversely affect your health. Also, it's a harsh but true fact: Alcohol shrinks your brain. If you value your brain cells, limit alcohol consumption.

11. DON'T SMOKE

Smoking constricts blood flow to your brain and prematurely ages it. Smoking is an extremely hazardous habit for people at high risk of stroke because certain chemicals found in cigarette smoke can affect the blood in such a way that it's more prone to clotting. In addition, nicotine damages the interior walls of blood vessels and makes them more susceptible to atherosclerosis. Numerous clinical studies have shown that our bodies begin repairing the damage to our respiratory system within days of that last cigarette. Unless you already have cancer or emphysema, the health of your lungs (and other organs adversely affected by tobacco, such as the heart) will continue to improve until, finally, you're almost as well as before you took that first puff.

12. LIMIT CAFFEINE

One of the world's most popular drugs, caffeine is a stimulant that affects the central nervous system, the digestive tract, and the metabolism. Caffeine is found in coffee beans, tea leaves, cocoa beans, and products derived from these sources. It is absorbed quickly in the body and can raise blood pressure, heart rate, and brain serotonin levels (low levels of serotonin cause drowsiness). Withdrawal from caffeine can cause headaches and drowsiness. The pharmacological active dose of caffeine is defined as 200 milligrams, and the daily recommended not-to-exceed intake level is the equivalent of one to three cups of coffee per day (139 to 417 milligrams). Too much caffeine also prematurely ages your brain because it dehydrates and reduces blood flow, and tricks you into thinking you don't need more sleep. Below is a guideline for approximate amounts of caffeine in commonly used foods and beverages:

Coffee, brewed from ground beans 6 oz	100 mg.
Coffee, instant 6 oz	65 mg.
Tea, brewed from whole leaves 6 oz	10–50 mg.
Cola, can or bottle 12 oz	50 mg.
Cocoa, breakfast type 6 oz	13 mg.
Cocoa, as milk chocolate bar 1 oz	6 mg.
Guarana, tablet or capsule 800 mg	30 mg.
Maté, brewed as tea 6 oz	25–50 mg.
One cup of semisweet chocolate chips	92 mg.
One cup of bittersweet chocolate chips	18–30 mg.
Caffeine tablet, proprietary product	100–200 mg.

APPROXIMATE AMOUNTS OF CAFFEINE IN COMMONLY USED FOODS & BEVERAGES

13. DON'T USE COFFEE AS A DRUG

According to the National Coffee Association, 80 percent of Americans drink coffee, and occasional coffee consumption rose 6 percent in the last year. At the same time, panic and other anxiety disorders have become the most common mental illnesses in the United States. Professionals agree that when caffeine overlaps with these disorders, the result can be trouble. Roland Griffiths,

PhD, a professor in the Departments of Psychiatry and Neuroscience at the Johns Hopkins University School of Medicine states, "Caffeine is the most widely used mood-altering drug in the world. People often see coffee, tea, and soft drinks simply as beverages rather than vehicles for a psychoactive drug. But caffeine can exacerbate anxiety and panic disorders."

14. KNOW YOUR RISK FOR HEART DISEASE

Heart disease is the leading killer of Americans today. Several risk factors are known to directly contribute to a higher risk of heart disease for both men and women; the more factors a person exhibits, the greater the risk. Risk factors include:

► Elevated cholesterol, especially with elevated LDL and low HDL
► Elevated triglycerides
► Smoking
► High blood pressure
► Diabetes
► Sedentary lifestyle
► Obesity, especially when the fat is concentrated above the waist area
► Stress
► Family history of heart disease
► Gender and age (risk starts earlier for men, increases for women post menopause)

You can reduce your risk by controlling all heart disease risk factors listed, except of course for family history, gender, and age.

15. REDUCE YOUR RISK OF HEART DISEASE

Several nutritional factors are important in helping to prevent heart disease. To reduce the impact of the controllable risk factors for heart disease, the American Heart Association (AHA) recommends the following population-wide dietary and lifestyle goals:

► Consume appropriate level of calories and perform physical activity.
► Eat a heart-healthy diet (specific information is available in *Feed Your Brain).*
► Eliminate cigarette smoking.
► Limit alcohol consumption to two drinks (1 to 2 ounces) per day.

Other recommendations include consuming at least 25 to 30 grams of fiber each day from sources such as whole grains, fruits, vegetables, and legumes. Consuming a variety of fruits and vegetables will also ensure that you receive plenty of beta carotene, vitamin C, folic acid, vitamin E, and other antioxidants and protective substances such as flavonoids and carotenoids. You can regularly add foods such as soy, oat bran, fish, nuts, seeds, and garlic to strengthen your disease-fighting prevention diet even more. Talk to your doctor about your risk for heart disease and how to manage any risk factors you may have.

16. EAT A HEART-HEALTHY DIET

The heart and blood vessels are responsible for transporting oxygen-rich and glucose-rich blood to all parts of the body. Impaired or damaged heart and blood vessels can't get enough oxygen or glucose to the brain. Coronary heart disease is easier to prevent than it is to treat, especially if you have a family history of heart problems. The keys to keeping coronary heart disease at bay are regular, heart-strengthening exercise (at least four times a week) and maintaining a healthful diet that is low in fat and cholesterol and high in antioxidant-rich fruits and vegetables. This book provides a lot of information on a heart-healthy diet in Chapters 4 and 5. Basically, a low-fat diet would have less animal protein, very little fried food, and increased amounts of whole grains and vegetables. Be good to your heart, and it will be good to your brain.

17. LIMIT HIGH-FAT FOODS

Improperly stored oils and fats will go rancid, and that's just what happens in the body when you eat a high-fat diet. Since the brain and nervous system are very high in fat, some researchers take the idea of rancid fat one step further and speculate that rancid fat may be damaging the brain by causing free radicals (unstable molecules that potentially cause cell damage). Scientists have discovered that eating a diet in which 40 percent of the calories come from fat raises the risk of Alzheimer's in someone who has the ApoE4 gene an incredible twenty-nine times. Younger people aged twenty to thirty-nine with the ApoE4 gene are twenty-three times more likely to develop Alzheimer's in later years than are healthy eaters.

18. DON'T SURRENDER ALL FATS

Each nerve cell in the brain is surrounded by a protective cell membrane. Receptors for many brain neurotransmitters are found on the membrane. This membrane is composed mostly of different types of fats, which include phosphatidylcholine (PC), also called lecithin; phosphatidylserine (PS); and phosphatidylethanolamine (PE). The function of the nerve cells and the neurotransmitters is highly dependent on the quality of fats that make up the cell membrane and therefore highly dependent on the type of fats and oils in your diet. The makeup of a cell membrane is always in a state of transition; it is constantly influenced by diet, stress, and the immune system. The bottom line: Your brain needs "good fats" like omega-3 fats, found in nuts, avocados and extra-virgin olive oil.

19. WATCH FOR CORRELATIONS

In 1969, elevated levels of an amino acid called homocysteine were found in the urine of patients with heart disease. Homocysteine is a normal by-product of protein digestion. If it occurs in elevated amounts it can cause cholesterol to change into an "oxidized," or rancid, form, which goes on to damage blood vessels. In the *New England Journal of Medicine* on February 14, 2002, the Boston University Medical Center reported on an eight-year study. In 1,092 patients, an increase in plasma homocysteine level of 5 umol/liter increased the risk of Alzheimer's disease by 40 percent. The highest levels doubled the risk. If various B vitamins (B_{12}, B_6, and folic acid) are deficient in your diet, homocysteine builds up. We'll address B vitamins in a later chapter. Just be aware that heart disease often correlates to brain dysfunction.

20. AVOID CHRONIC STRESS

Researchers at the James A. Haley Veterans Administration Medical Center, at the University of South Florida (USF), and Arizona State University (ASU) found that chronically stressed rats consuming an "American-style" diet of excessive carbohydrates and beef fat developed atrophy in the hippocampus, the part of the brain that is essential for learning and remembering new information. Rats fed a high-fat diet and living under chronic stress (living in crowded conditions, in close proximity to cats) developed hippocampal atrophy, expressed in reduced dendrite length. Dendrites are the connections between brain cells where information is stored. The researchers deduced that the combination of a high-fat diet and stress can interfere with the ability of the brain—in rats or people—to learn new information. Previous research had shown that rats on a high-fat diet produce an excessive amount of corticosterone in response to stress. Corticosterone, a steroid hormone produced by the adrenal glands, can also damage the hippocampus, indicating that a high-fat diet and stress are doubly detrimental to the brain.

21. UNDERSTAND FREE RADICALS

Free radicals are unbalanced oxygen molecules containing an extra electron. Because nature likes equilibrium, free radicals are constantly searching for molecules to which they can attach and steal a matching electron. However, the theft of a matching electron only serves to create new free radicals in an ongoing process that ultimately results in cellular damage. It's important to note, however, that free radical activity—a form of biochemical electricity—is not in itself bad. Without it, a great many important bodily functions, including hormone synthesis, smooth-muscle tone, and the maintenance of a strong immune system, would cease. Problems occur when free radicals attack cell membranes, inhibiting the cells' ability to reproduce or protect themselves. The effects of too many free radicals include signs of aging, including wrinkles, age spots, and poor skin quality; an abundance can also lead to more serious problems, including cataracts, heart disease, and certain kinds of cancer. Anti-aging researchers say that the answer can be found in chemicals known as antioxidants, which eat up excess free radicals.

22. GET THOSE RADICALS UNDER CONTROL

Free radicals age your brain. A free radical is an unstable molecule that is formed when molecules within the body's cells react with oxygen. It is unstable because it has an unpaired electron that steals a stabilizing electron from another molecule, potentially causing cell damage. The body's own metabolism causes free radicals, but there are also external sources, i.e., pollution. Antioxidants are vitamins and minerals such as magnesium, selenium, vitamin C, and vitamin E stored in the body whose job it is to neutralize free radicals, but if there aren't enough antioxidants available, excess free radicals begin to damage and destroy normal healthy cells, leading to degenerative diseases. They can damage any body structure by affecting proteins, enzymes, fats, and even DNA. Free radicals are implicated in more than sixty different health conditions, including Alzheimer's, heart disease, autoimmune diseases, and cancer. Vitamins C and E are natural antioxidants that may clean up roving free radicals before they inflict damage on the brain.

23. BE PRO-ANTIOXIDANTS

With aging, the body's stores of antioxidants become lowered unless they are regularly replenished with an excellent diet or supplements. Free radicals can build up in all parts of the body, including the brain. When they enter nerve cells they can disrupt function and cause cell death. They can also trigger a cascade of free radical formation. This chain reaction can cause widespread oxidative damage in the brain. The avenues of research regarding Alzheimer's and antioxidants, in the form of comprehensive dietary surveys and laboratory studies, suggest that low-fat, low-calorie diets and certain supplements may be beneficial in Alzheimer's treatment.

24. UNDERSTAND STROKES

Stroke is a medical condition characterized by sudden or gradual neurological impairment resulting from reduced blood flow to the brain and the subsequent death of brain cells that are dependent on blood for oxygen. Brain cells are very sensitive and begin to starve when deprived of oxygen for even a few minutes. Prolonged oxygen deprivation usually results in permanent brain damage. Sometimes referred to as a "brain attack," stroke is the third leading cause of death in the United States, behind heart disease and cancer. An estimated 500,000 Americans experience a new or recurrent stroke every year, and nearly a third of cases are fatal. Risk of stroke increases dramatically after age fifty-five. Common risk factors include poorly managed hypertension (high blood pressure), a family history of stroke, a personal history of "mini-strokes," known as transient ischemic attacks (TIAs), atherosclerosis (particularly in the neck, heart, and legs), atrial fibrillation, and a history of smoking.

25. KNOW YOUR RISK FOR STROKE

Stroke is usually caused by a blood clot or buildup of cholesterol plaque that blocks an artery in the brain. Depending on where it occurs, it can mimic any and all symptoms of dementia. The incidence of stroke is about four out of 1,000 people; it is the third leading cause of death in the United States. Risk for stroke includes high blood pressure, heart disease, smoking, high cholesterol, and diabetes. If you have a high risk for stroke, it's extremely important that you take concrete steps to safeguard your brain from this type of devastating blow.

26. REDUCE YOUR RISK OF STROKE

Current research, from a long-term study on Alzheimer's and aging, seems to suggest that a stroke can be a significant risk factor for Alzheimer's. It appears that even without an abundance of plaques and tangles (abnormal deposits in brain cells) the brain of a stroke patient is susceptible to the ravages of Alzheimer's.

Researchers are intrigued by the Alzheimer's-stroke connection because stroke is very common and a major cause of death in our society. With new research on lifestyle intervention, we can modify the risk factors for stroke, lower the stroke rate, and thereby decrease the incidence of Alzheimer's in this group. Stroke risk factors include hypertension, high cholesterol, and smoking. Any measures you take to reduce your risk of stroke will benefit your brain in multiple ways.

27. UNDERSTAND ALZHEIMER'S

Today, late-onset Alzheimer's disease is known to be the most common cause of loss of mental function in people over sixty-five. Approximately 4 million Americans are believed to have Alzheimer's disease, 90 percent of them over age sixty. The brains of Alzheimer's patients contain distinctive, abnormally shaped proteins known as tangles and plaques. Tangles are long, silk-like tendrils found inside neurons. Plaques are clumps of silk-like fibers that typically form outside the neurons in adjacent brain tissue. The areas most commonly afflicted by tangles and plaques are related to memory. In the 1980s, researchers found that a compound in plaques, known as amyloid protein, may actually be poisonous to brain cells. And more recent research suggests that a protein called tau may be responsible for the telltale tangles found in the brains of Alzheimer's patients. In healthy brains, tau gives neurons structural support, but in Alzheimer's patients, this structural support collapses into useless twists and tangles.

28. LIMIT MERCURY IN YOUR DIET

Research has shown that nerve cells exposed to mercury caused the formation of neurofibrillar tangles and amyloid plaques, often present in Alzheimer's cases. Dr. Haley, a Canadian researcher, said, "Seven of the characteristic markers that we look for to distinguish Alzheimer's disease can be produced in normal brain tissues, or cultures of neurons, by the addition of extremely low levels of mercury. In addition, research [in 1998] has shown that Alzheimer's diseased patients have at least three times higher blood levels of mercury than controls" (*NeuroReport*, 12[4]: 733–737, 2001). Dr. William R. Markesbery, director of the Sanders-Brown Center on Aging at the University of Kentucky, found in 1990 that the Alzheimer's patients' brain tissue had almost double the concentration of mercury as that of patients who died of all other causes. One particular area of the brain that transmits memories and sensations to higher brain centers contained almost four times as much mercury as did the normal controls. We'll discuss high and low mercury fish in Chapter 4.

29. DON'T REST ON YOUR LAURELS

Most adults are all at Stage 1 Alzheimer's, with no noticeable symptoms. Sixty percent of the general population has the ApoE4 gene that creates a susceptibility to Alzheimer's. Many of us are at risk for stroke or have high levels of homocysteine, which also increases our risk for Alzheimer's. This is the stage where lifestyle intervention, in the form of a good diet, exercise, and certain nutrients, could mean the difference between health and Alzheimer's. This is the stage in the brain where plaques and tangles could start to build up, but take ten to twenty years to be recognized as impaired memory.

30. BOOST YOUR METABOLISM

All activity in the body occurs through a process called metabolism in which cells break down chemicals and nutrients to generate energy and form new molecules like proteins. Efficient metabolism requires blood loaded with oxygen, glucose, and nutrients. Enzymes are the molecules that make metabolism happen, and nutrients are vitamins and minerals that act as essential co-enzymes. When a nutrient is deficient in the body, certain metabolic functions are impeded and symptoms of disease can arise. Eat a healthy diet, add exercise, and keep your body in top running form, and it will nourish your brain.

31. GET PLENTY OF SLEEP

Your body, including your brain, actually mends and maintains itself when you sleep. If you strength train or do any sort of resistance exercise, then your muscles repair themselves and grow stronger when you're asleep. If you don't sleep, your muscles will stay fatigued and not get stronger. Getting enough sleep helps keep you safe; being sleep-deprived increases the likelihood of accidents and mistakes. It's helpful to first recognize that you want to sleep well, i.e., seven to nine hours of uninterrupted sleep each night. Go to sleep and wake up at the same times. Your body loves regularity. If you are someone who sleeps very late on the weekends and then has trouble waking up for work on Monday, or if you sometimes stay up late and then crash the next evening, you aren't helping yourself. Instead, seek regularity in your sleeping patterns.

32. WEAR A HELMET

When you fall and hit your head and go unconscious, even though you can't see through your skull, you are likely bruised and bleeding. We now know that if you are unconscious for over an hour from a head injury, you have twice the risk of developing Alzheimer's. After the bleeding stops and the swelling goes down after head trauma, you can still have scar tissue that may be involved in the future development of Alzheimer's. Also, it's been estimated that 75 percent of all bicycling deaths result from brain injury. It's imperative that you wear a helmet when riding a motorcycle, but skateboarding, bicycling, hockey, football, and rock climbing are all sports that encourage participants to wear helmets. If you even suspect that your brain might be susceptible to injury, forgo cool and strap on a helmet. ✳

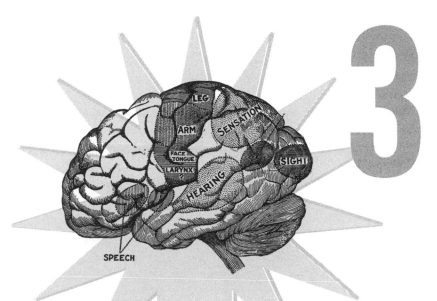

SPEECH

3

FEED
YOUR BRAIN—
BASICS

23

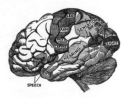

FEED YOUR BRAIN— BASICS

Nutrition plays an essential role in our overall health and longevity.

33. UNDERSTAND MACRONUTRIENTS

The brain is only a fraction of the total weight of the body, about 2 percent, but requires 20 percent of the body's blood supply, 20 percent of the body's total oxygen supply, and 65 percent of its glucose. Along with the rich supply of glucose comes a host of nutrients that are needed by the brain. Nutrients are grouped into six different categories: carbohydrates, proteins, fats, vitamins, minerals, and water. Carbohydrates, proteins, and fats are called macronutrients because we need larger amounts in our diet. Some foods consist of one, two, or all three of these macronutrients. Even though each macronutrient has a particular function in the body, they work in partnership for good health. Our bodies need all three macronutrients to function properly, but not in equal amounts. Some evidence suggests that a diet with macronutrients in the wrong proportions is a risk factor for diseases like coronary heart disease and certain cancers.

34. MAKE NUTRITION A PRIORITY

Nutrition, perhaps more than any other factor, plays an essential role in our over-all health and longevity. The reason for this is simple: The foods we eat affect virtually every cell, organ, and system in our bodies. If we eat enough of the right foods, our bodies thrive, and we live well and long. According to nutrition experts, a healthful diet provides our cells with everything they need to function well, reproduce, and repair damage from a variety of sources. Healthful foods also give our bodies the right kind of fuel so that we have plenty of energy and a strong immune system. But there's more. The right kinds of foods help our bodies get rid of waste products and potentially harmful toxins, many of which can increase our risk of serious illness, including cancer, if not purged regularly. And they help reduce our risk of many chronic disorders commonly associated with aging, including osteoporosis and heart disease.

35. FRESHEN UP YOUR ATTITUDE

The harmful effects of a poor diet—that is, too much red meat and fried, fatty foods and too few fruits and vegetables—are almost too numerous to count. A lousy diet can be a springboard for a wide variety of age-related problems, including atherosclerosis, hypertension, heart disease, diabetes, osteoporosis, a weakened immune response, and even cancer. But a simple change in dietary habits can have a remarkable effect on your health and, in turn, how you age—no matter how old you are when you start. For most people, simply eating less red meat and fatty foods and more fresh vegetables and fruits improves their health. This reduces the amount of cholesterol in your system, gives your body the vitamins and minerals it needs to function well, and packs your system with antioxidants and other anti-aging compounds.

36. MAKE HEALTHY FOOD CHOICES

Here's reality: Some foods are very good for your body (and your brain); some are not. We'll go over choices in greater detail in Chapter 4, but the basics come down to the following:

Food that improves your health:

► Omega-3 fatty acids found in fish, flax oil, and spinach
► Colorful vegetables that are rich in antioxidants
► Whole foods such as brown rice, whole wheat bread and pasta, and legumes
► Clean protein from organic meats, fish, soy, and legumes

Food that has an adverse effect on your health:

► Excess saturated fat (meat, cheese, and fried food)
► Trans fat (margarines, baked goods, chips, and fast food)
► High-calorie food
► Refined carbohydrates like white rice, white bread, chips, pasta, and cookies

37. FOLLOW AMERICAN HEART ASSOCIATION GUIDELINES

The American Heart Association's dietary guidelines provide useful parameters for optimum health.

► Dietary fat intake should be less than 30 percent of total calories.
► Saturated fat intake should be less than 10 percent of total calories.
► Polyunsaturated fat should not exceed 10 percent of total calories.
► Cholesterol intake should not exceed 300 milligrams per day.

- ► Carbohydrate intake should represent 50 percent or more total calories with emphasis on complex carbohydrates.
- ► Protein intake should constitute the remainder of the calories.
- ► Sodium intake should be limited to less than 3 grams per day.
- ► Alcohol consumption is not recommended, but if consumed, it should not exceed 1 ounce a day of hard liquor, 8 ounces of wine, or 24 ounces of beer.

38. PROPORTION YOUR DIET

Don't count grams of nutrients. Instead, think about your meals. Here's the ideal proportion of your food intake: Get 50 percent of your calories from carbs, 30 percent from protein, and 20 percent from fat—the pounds will come off without your doing any other counting.

39. KNOW THE FACTS ABOUT SUGAR

The typical American diet is packed with sugar, and most of it is hidden. Nutrition experts agree that Americans need to cut back. There is no current RDA for sugar, but experts recommend that about 55 to 60 percent of total calories in your diet should come from carbohydrates, with less than 10 percent coming from simple sugars. The bulk of carbohydrate choices should be complex carbohydrates, and most of the simple carbohydrate choices should come from fruits and dairy products, which also contain vitamins, minerals, and fiber. The USDA advises people who eat a 2,000-calorie healthful diet to try to limit themselves to about 10 teaspoons (40 grams) of added sugars per day.

40. LIMIT SIMPLE SUGARS

Sugars are simple carbohydrates that the body uses as a source of energy. During digestion, all carbohydrates break down into sugar, or blood glucose. Some sugars occur naturally, such as in dairy products (as lactose) and fruits (as fructose). Other foods have added sugars, or sugar that is added in processing or preparation. The body cannot tell the difference between naturally occurring sugar and added sugar. Most foods containing added sugars provide calories but little in the way of essential nutrients such as fiber, vitamins, and minerals. Sugar can be part of a healthy diet if consumed in moderation.

41. KNOW WHEN YOU'RE CONSUMING WAY TOO MUCH SUGAR

Individual foods provide large fractions of the USDA's recommended sugar limits. For instance, a cup of regular ice cream provides 60 percent of a day's worth of added sugar, a 12-ounce Pepsi provides 103 percent, and a Hostess Lemon Fruit Pie provides 115 percent. Carbohydrates are broken down into glucose and used as energy. They are also stored in the muscles and liver as glycogen. When too many sugar calories are consumed, they may be converted to body fat. Avoiding sugars alone will not correct a weight problem. When trying to lose weight, reduce the total amount of calories from the food you eat and increase your level of physical activity.

42. EAT BREAKFAST

Breakfast is one of the most important meals, yet it is probably the most skipped meal of the day. The word *breakfast* describes exactly what it does: breaks a fast. After a good night's rest, your body has gone eight to twelve hours without food or energy. Blood sugar, or glucose, which comes from the breakdown of food in the body, is your body's main source of energy. Eating food provides your body with a fresh supply of blood glucose or energy. The brain in particular needs a fresh supply of glucose each day because that is its main source of energy. (The brain does not store glucose.) Eating breakfast is associated with being more productive and efficient in the morning hours. Breakfast eaters tend to experience better concentration, problem-solving ability, strength, and endurance. Your muscles also rely on a fresh supply of blood glucose for physical activity throughout the day. Here are a few healthy suggestions:

► Cold cereal with fruit and skim milk
► Bran muffin and a banana
► Hard-boiled egg and grapefruit juice
► Yogurt with fruit or low-fat granola cereal
► Peanut butter on a whole-wheat bagel and orange juice
► Instant oatmeal with raisins or berries
► Breakfast smoothie (blend fruit and skim milk)
► Cottage cheese and peaches

43. EAT BREAKFAST TO LOSE WEIGHT

Do you think that eating breakfast might make you gain weight? Eating a good healthy breakfast can help regulate your appetite throughout the day. Breakfast can help you eat in moderation at lunch and dinner. Also, research indicates that a high-fiber, low-fat breakfast may make a major contribution to a total reduced fat intake for the day. If you have a hard time facing food first thing in the morning, start with eating a light breakfast, such as a piece of toast or fruit. Pack a breakfast or snack to take with you so you can eat once you do get hungry.

44. DON'T SKIP MEALS

You need to fuel your body throughout the day with nutritious foods for optimal energy and performance. Skipping meals can have numerous negative effects on your healthy lifestyle. Skipping meals can make you so hungry that you overeat at your next eating opportunity, and likely won't eat as healthily either. Skipping meals can negatively affect your productivity, concentration, and energy level throughout the day. Finally, skipping meals increases the chance that you will not consume all of your needed servings from the USDA's MyPyramid (covered in Chapter 4). So make time and even schedule eating opportunities throughout the day.

45. EYEBALL PROPORTIONS

To follow a healthy diet, you don't need to weigh and measure all of your food each day. Keep in mind that portion sizes are meant as general guidelines, so the aim is to come close to the recommended serving sizes, on average, over several days. Use these visual comparisons to help estimate your portion sizes:

▶ A 3-ounce portion of cooked meat, poultry, or fish is about the size of a deck of playing cards.

▶ A medium potato is about the size of a computer mouse.

▶ 1 cup of rice or pasta is about the size of a fist or a tennis ball.

▶ A cup of fruit or a medium apple or orange is the size of a baseball.

▶ ½ cup of chopped vegetables is about the size of three regular ice cubes.

▶ 3 ounces of grilled fish is the size of your checkbook.

▶ 1 ounce of cheese is the size of four dice.

▶ 1 teaspoon of peanut butter equals one die; 2 tablespoons is about the size of a golf ball.

▶ 1 ounce of snack foods—pretzels, etc.—equals a large handful.

▶ 1 thumb tip equals 1 teaspoon; 3 thumb tips equal 1 tablespoon; and a whole thumb equals 1 ounce.

46. SLOW DOWN!

It takes at least twenty minutes for your stomach to signal your brain that it is full. Slowing down will help to curb the urge to go back for a second helping. It also ensures proper digestion. To slow down, between bites take sips of your beverage, put your fork down, and enjoy the conversation of others. Sit down to eat instead of eating while standing, driving, or watching television. Eating while doing other things means you are eating unconsciously, and easily consume more.

47. DISTINGUISH BETWEEN HUNGER AND CRAVINGS

The question is, is it a craving, or am I really hungry? Hunger signals are your stomach's way of informing you that it is empty or your brain's way of informing you that it is lacking an energy supply. Signals from your stomach may include growls, pangs, or hollow feelings. Signals from your brain may include fogginess, lack of concentration, headache, or fatigue. Cravings can be caused by either physical or psychological needs. Giving in to too many cravings can lead to overeating, unhealthy eating, and extra weight gain. Healthy eating means eating when you are truly hungry and eating until you are satisfied.

48. KNOW YOUR CHOLESTEROL NUMBERS

It is important to ask your doctor for a total lipoprotein profile so that you are aware of not only your total cholesterol but of each component of your cholesterol. You may have a total cholesterol level that is desirable, but that doesn't mean your HDL and LDL levels are in line. Your total cholesterol level will fall into one of three categories:

- Desirable: less than 200 mg/dL
- Borderline high risk: 200–239 mg/dL
- High risk: 240 mg/dL and over

If you fall within the borderline high-risk range, you have at least twice the risk of a heart attack compared with someone who is in the desirable range.

49. TAKE HIGH CHOLESTEROL VERY SERIOUSLY

If you have a cholesterol reading over 240 mg/dL or you have risk factors such as heart disease along with cholesterol readings over 200 mg/dL, your doctor will probably prescribe a cholesterol-lowering medication in combination with a healthy low-fat diet and exercise. Your doctor should periodically test your blood cholesterol levels to check on your progress.

50. WORK TO LOWER YOUR LDL AND RAISE YOUR HDL

The bottom line is that the less LDL you have, and the more HDL, or good cholesterol, you have, the lower your risk for heart disease. When it comes to trying to lower your LDL, food choices are key. A combination of a diet low in saturated fat and cholesterol, regular physical activity, and a healthy weight can help you lower your total cholesterol as well as raise your HDL, lower your LDL, and lower your triglycerides. It is important to focus on your cholesterol intake as well as your saturated fat intake, which often occur together in foods. Cholesterol and most saturated fats come *only* from animal foods. Even though some foods of plant origin are high in fat or saturated fat, all plant foods are cholesterol-free. Nuts, for example, are high in fat—mostly unsaturated fat—but are cholesterol-free.

51. MINIMIZE FOODS HIGH IN LDL

We get cholesterol in two ways. The body, mainly the liver, produces varying amounts of cholesterol each day. Cholesterol also comes directly from animal foods such as egg yolks, meat, poultry, fish, seafood, and whole-milk dairy products. Typically our body makes all the cholesterol it needs, so we don't need to consume it. Saturated fat raises your LDL-cholesterol level more than anything else in the diet. Trans fats also raise blood cholesterol, as well as dietary cholesterol itself. The American Heart Association recommends that you "limit your average daily cholesterol intake to less than 300 mg. If you have heart disease, limit your daily intake to less than 200 mg." Foods high in saturated fat generally contain substantial amounts of dietary cholesterol. Here are a few ways you can lower LDL in your diet:

► Buy lower-fat versions of fats such as dressings, mayonnaise, margarine, and cream cheese.
► Eat no more than four egg yolks per week. Egg yolks contain about 215 mg from a large egg, but the egg white has *no* cholesterol. Try substituting two egg whites for one whole egg in baked goods or using an egg substitute.
► Limit organ meats such as liver. They are nutritious but also very high in cholesterol.
► Enjoy seafood, prepared in a low-fat way, as your main meal a few times per week.
► Make vegetarian meals occasionally. Meals with beans or soy products as the main protein source have several cholesterol-lowering qualities.

52. SWITCH FROM BUTTER TO CHOLESTEROL-LOWERING MARGARINES

Various margarines on the market today are low in both saturated fats and trans fatty acids. Trans fatty acids are created through the process of hydrogenation. They can increase LDL cholesterol and lower HDL. Many of these margarines are called "spreads" because they are less than 80 percent oil. The more solid a margarine is, the more saturated fat and trans fat they contain. When looking for margarine spreads, look for a margarine spread with no more than 30 percent fat from saturated plus trans fat. Less than 20 percent is even better. Also, look for words such as *trans-free*, which means the spread has no more than half a gram of trans fat per serving. But be sure they are not replacing trans fats with saturated fats. These new margarine spreads are not a magic bullet to lowering cholesterol, but in moderation they can be part of your heart-healthy lifestyle.

53. SNACK SMARTLY

Contrary to popular belief, snacking can be part of a healthful eating plan. Choosing snacks wisely can help fuel your body between meals, give you an energy boost, and add to your total intake of essential nutrients for the day. Snacking can also help to take the edge off hunger between meals. The longer you wait between meals, the more you tend to eat at the next meal. Leaving only about three to four hours between meals is an ideal amount of time to keep blood sugar levels in control. The key to smart snacking is the type and amounts of food that you choose.

► Choose snacks that are lower in fat and nutrient-rich.
► Plan and eat snacks well ahead of mealtime.
► Make snacks part of your eating plan for the day instead of thinking of them as an extra.

- ► Make snacking a conscious activity.
- ► Eat smaller portion snacks, not meal-size ones.

54. CHOOSE HEALTHY SNACKS

Try some of these smart snacks as part of your healthy eating plan:

- ► Half a bagel with peanut butter
- ► Raw vegetables with low-fat or fat-free dressing
- ► Fruit yogurt topped with low-fat granola cereal
- ► Low-fat cottage cheese topped with fresh fruit
- ► Fresh fruit
- ► Light microwave popcorn
- ► Pita bread stuffed with fresh veggies and low-fat dressing
- ► Low-fat string cheese
- ► Whole-grain cereal and fat-free milk
- ► Vegetable juice

55. STAY HYDRATED

Simple dehydration can cause the brain to react in strange ways. Fogginess, dizziness, and lack of concentration are all symptoms of dehydration. Water is one of the most abundant substances in your body and is the nutrient your body needs in the greatest amounts. Almost 55 to 75 percent of an adult's body weight is water. Water is present in every part of your body: It comprises 83 percent of blood, 73 percent of muscle, 25 percent of body fat, and even 22 percent of bones. Water plays a vital role in almost every major function in the body. Water helps to regulate body temperature through perspiration. It transports nutrients and oxygen through the body, carries waste products away from the body cells, cushions joints, and protects body organs. Water is the solution in which all other nutrients are dissolved. It serves as a shock absorber inside the eyes and spinal cord. This amazing nutrient also moistens body tissues in your eyes, mouth, and nose. Water is vital to the digestive process: Some of the water in your body comes from the breakdown or metabolism of carbohydrates, proteins, and fats. Water also helps soften the stool to prevent constipation.

56. KNOW HOW MUCH WATER YOU NEED

The body has no provision to store water. Therefore, the amount of water lost each day must be continually replaced to maintain good health and proper body function. On average, we lose about 10 cups of water each day just through perspiration, breathing, urination, and bowel movements. This does not include hot days or exercise when you perspire even more. The average adult needs 8 to 12 cups of water each day. To avoid dehydration, the body needs an ongoing supply of water throughout the day. By the time you feel thirsty, you can already be on your way to becoming dehydrated. To be sure you are properly hydrated, check your urine to make sure it is clear (meaning diluted) rather than a darker yellow.

57. LOAD UP ON PHYTONUTRIENTS

Phyto is the Greek word for "plant"; phytonutrients are the vitamins and minerals derived from fruits and vegetables. Phytonutrients flush toxic chemicals from our bodies, inhibit free-radical damage, and keep certain hormones, such as estrogen, at optimal levels. Think of them as nature's pharmacy—free, safe, and readily available. The various types are as follows:

Allylic sulfides. These compounds give onions, garlic, and related herbs their pungent odor and unique flavor. They raise HDL cholesterol (the so-called "good cholesterol"), lower blood triglyceride levels, protect the heart, and stimulate the production of enzymes believed to suppress the growth of certain types of tumors.

Carotenoids. These compounds are found in abundance in carrots, broccoli, cantaloupe, cauliflower, green leafy vegetables, and tomatoes. They are powerful antioxidants and play an instrumental role in preventing heart disease and certain forms of cancer.

Flavonoids. Also members of the antioxidant family, these chemicals can be found in apples, citrus fruit, cranberries, endive, grape juice, kale, onions, and red wine. Their primary benefit is the prevention of heart disease and blood clots.

Indoles and isothiocyanates. These compounds are plentiful in broccoli, cabbage, cauliflower, and mustard greens. They help stimulate enzymes known to prevent cancer and block estrogen activity in cells.

Isoflavones. These chemicals, which also prevent the formation of certain cancers and block estrogen activity in the cells, can be found in chickpeas, kidney beans, lentils, and soybeans.

Lignans. These chemicals are known antioxidants and block estrogen activity in the cells as well as help prevent the formation of certain cancers. They are particularly abundant in flaxseed.

Monoterpenes. Yet another cancer preventative, this phytonutrient blocks the action of certain cancer-causing compounds. It can be found in citrus fruits such as oranges and grapefruit, as well as cherries.

Phenolic compounds. These antioxidants help activate important cancer-fighting enzymes. To add them to your diet, eat plenty of fruit, vegetables, and cereal grains, and drink green or black teas.

Saponins. These chemicals bind with cholesterol and help the body flush it out. They also stimulate the immune system and help prevent heart disease and certain types of cancer. They can be found in chickpeas, nuts, oats, potatoes, soybeans, spinach, and tomatoes.

58. BULK UP WITH FIBER
Nutritionally speaking, fiber is the indigestible part of the food we eat—the stuff that passes through our digestive system relatively quickly and intact, such as the bran in grain, the pulp in fruit, and the skin of certain vegetables such as corn. By traveling so quickly, it also rushes other foods through our system, giving cancer-causing compounds less time to do their dirty work. It is also believed that fiber dilutes potential carcinogens, reducing their ability to do harm. And fiber also promotes healthy digestion by stimulating the action of beneficial bacteria.

59. KNOW YOUR LIMITS
Are you getting enough fiber in your diet? Despite efforts by government health agencies to boost fiber intake, the typical American still consumes an average of only 11 grams a day. According to the National Cancer Institute, an amount double that would be far more healthful. Studies have shown that consuming between

20 and 30 grams of fiber a day can dramatically reduce your risk of many cancers. Consuming more than that, however, can cause painful and embarrassing bloating and flatulence. To avoid these problems, you should introduce fiber into your diet gradually and try to get as much as you can from the foods you eat, rather than relying on fiber supplements.

60. KNOW YOUR FIBERS

There are four major types of fiber, each of which can benefit your body in a special way:

- ► *Cellulose.* This is the most common type of fiber and is found in most fruits and vegetables, as well as whole grains and some types of nuts. Cellulose is an effective stool softener and helps dilute bile acids in the colon, which are believed to stimulate the growth of certain types of cancer.
- ► *Gums.* These are sticky fibers derived from plants. They help lower cholesterol and prevent certain types of cancer, though researchers are still trying to figure out exactly how they work. Gums are found in oat bran, dried beans, and oatmeal and are commonly used to thicken processed foods.
- ► *Lignin.* This fiber acts as a binder for cellulose and is found in certain fruits, nuts, peas, tomatoes, and whole grains. It doesn't have the same action as cellulose on stools or bile acids, but laboratory studies have shown that it can help prevent the onset of cancer.
- ► *Pectin.* This gelatinous compound supplements the action of cellulose. It helps limit the potential damage from bile acids and also aids digestion by preventing diarrhea. Rich sources of pectin include apples, bananas, beets, carrots, and a wide array of citrus fruit.

61. INCREASE FIBER IN YOUR DIET

Adding fiber to your diet may be easier than you think. Here are some tips that can help you get started:

▶ Look at the fiber content on the Nutrition Facts Label on packaged foods. Good sources of fiber have at least 2.5 grams of fiber per serving.

▶ Substitute higher fiber foods, such as whole-grain breads, brown rice, whole-wheat pasta, and fruits and vegetables, for lower fiber foods, such as white bread, white rice, candy, and chips.

▶ Eat more raw vegetables and fresh fruits, and include the skins when appropriate. Cooking vegetables can reduce their fiber content, and skins are a good source of fiber.

▶ Plan to eat high-fiber foods such as fruits, vegetables, legumes, or whole-grain starches at every meal.

▶ Start your day with a high-fiber breakfast cereal, such as bran cereal or oatmeal. Look for cereals that contain at least 5 grams of fiber per serving. Add fresh fruit for an extra fiber boost.

▶ Eat a variety of high-fiber foods to ensure you get a mix of both types of fiber.

▶ Use snacks to increase your fiber intake by nibbling on higher fiber foods, such as dried fruits, popcorn, fresh fruit, raw vegetables, or whole-wheat crackers.

▶ Try to eat legumes, or dried beans, at least two to three times per week. Add them to salads, soups, casseroles, or spaghetti sauce.

▶ Eat whole fruits more often than juice. Most of the fiber in fruit is found in the skin and pulp, which is removed when the juice is made.

62. SOW YOUR OATS

Oats are a marvelous source of energy, and oat bran is an excellent fiber that can reduce serum cholesterol. An oat extract can be used to relieve indigestion (10 to 20 drops up to 3 times daily). Used in the bath, oats are soothing to the skin and calming to the psyche.

63. ADD OAT BRAN TO YOUR DIET

Keep in mind that you need to eat more oats and oatmeal than oat bran, which is concentrated. Oat bran that is removed from the whole oat is sold in the cereal aisle of the supermarket, alongside the oatmeal, and in health food stores. Try sprinkling oat bran on cereal and yogurt. Add it to toppings for fruit crisps and casseroles. Use it to coat chicken, lean meats, or fish before baking, or add it to meat loaf or meatballs in place of some of the breadcrumbs.

64. LOVE THOSE OMEGAS

Preliminary research indicates that omega-3 fatty acids may decrease the risk of stroke and heart attack. Omega-3 fatty acids may also protect against arrhythmias (abnormal heart rhythms), the leading cause of death after heart attacks. Omega-3 fatty acids may provide protection by enhancing the stability of the heart cells and increasing their resistance to becoming overexcited. In the Physicians' Health Study, those who ate fish just one to two times per week had a 40 percent reduction in sudden deaths from cardiac arrhythmias. Foods rich in omega-3 fatty acids include dried butternuts, black walnuts, raw (green) soybeans, sardines, lake trout, Chinook salmon, and cooked pinto beans.

65. USE OMEGAS TO STABILIZE MOOD SWINGS

Preliminary but exciting new research suggests that omega-3 fatty acids may help decrease symptoms of bipolar disorder (or manic depression). Researchers at Harvard University suggest that omega-3 fats may interfere with the brain signals that trigger the characteristic mood swings seen with bipolar disorder. Interestingly, the investigators reported unusually high patient interest and acceptance of omega-3 fatty acids as mood stabilizers. The supplements were viewed as "natural" compounds with few side effects. If these findings hold true in future studies, omega-3 fatty acids may have implications for treating other psychiatric disorders such as depression and schizophrenia. Try taking at least 10 grams of fish oil a day to see if it helps with mood stabilization. If you have been diagnosed as bipolar, do not substitute fish oil for your medication.

66. EAT FISH LOW IN MERCURY CONTENT

Fish is high in omega-3 oils so it's very healthy to eat fish, but some fish is higher in mercury content. The FDA and EPA recommend limited consumption of shark, swordfish, king mackerel, or tilefish because they contain high levels of mercury. They also recommend no more than 6 oz (170 g) per week of canned albacore ("white") tuna, tuna steaks, lobster, halibut, and orange roughy. A 6-ounce serving is about the size of two decks of cards or two checkbooks. The FDA also recommends that you eat no more than 12 oz (340 g) per week of fish and shellfish lower in mercury. This equates to two average 6 oz (170 g) meals. Fish lower in mercury include shrimp, canned light tuna (not albacore tuna), salmon, pollock, and catfish, cod, crab, flounder/sole, grouper, haddock, herring, mahi-mahi, ocean perch, oysters, rainbow trout, sardines, scallops, shrimp, tilapia, and trout.

67. CUT BACK ON BRAIN DRAINS

Cut down on alcohol, sugar, aspartame sweetener, and MSG. They all interfere with brain function. Alcohol makes you dull; sugar makes you foggy; aspartame and MSG are brain excitotoxins and can lead to brain cell death.

68. AVOID SODA

The brain uses 65 percent of the body's glucose, but too much or too little glucose can have a detrimental effect on brain function. When you drink a can of soda, which contains ten teaspoons of table sugar, that sugar is absorbed into a blood-stream that only contains a total of four teaspoons of blood sugar. The blood sugar level rockets to an excessive level, setting off alarms in the pancreas, and a large amount of insulin comes out to deal with the excess blood sugar. Some sugar is quickly ushered into the cells, including brain cells, and the rest is put into storage or into fat cells. When all this is done, maybe in about one hour, the blood sugar may fall dramatically and low blood sugar occurs. These rapid swings in blood sugar produce symptoms of impaired memory and clouded thinking. ✳

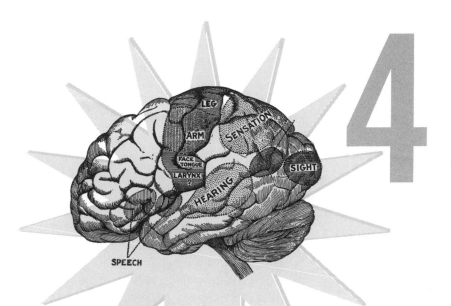

FEED YOUR BRAIN— GUIDELINES

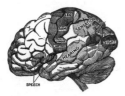

FEED YOUR BRAIN— GUIDELINES

Balancing what we eat is important for our mental health.

69. FOLLOW THE USDA MyPyramid GUIDELINES

In 2005, the USDA replaced the Food Guide Pyramid with MyPyramid, symbolizing a personalized apporach to healthy eating and physical activity. It gives the guidance you need to recognize what and how much to eat of each of five major food groups daily. Following MyPyramid will help you keep your fat intake at recommended levels and help you consume all the essential nutrients that make up a healthy diet. The pyramid conveys three messages: variety, balance, and moderation. Eating a variety of foods ensures that you meet your nutritional requirements and also provides a much wider variety of nutrients to your diet. Balancing the food groups in your diet also provides variety and supplies a better balance of nutrients. To eat in moderation, choose the number of servings that meet your calorie needs and limit the total amount of fat, cholesterol, sodium, sugar, and alcoholic beverages you consume. The food groups in the pyramid include the following:

- Grains
- Vegetables
- Fruits
- Milk
- Meat and beans
- Oils

70. CHOOSE COMPLEX CARBOHYDRATES

Carbohydrates are your body's main source of energy, especially for the brain and nervous system. Carbohydrates are found in fruits, vegetables, dairy products, starches, and foods in the meat group such as beans and soy products. The only food they are not found in is meat. Carbohydrates are either simple carbohydrates (sugars) or complex carbohydrates (starches). Sugars are carbohydrates in their simplest form. Refined sugars are found in table sugar, honey, jams, candy, syrup, and soft drinks, all of which lack vitamins, minerals, and fiber. Some simple sugars, such as naturally occurring sugars, are found in more nutritious foods, such as fructose found in fruit and lactose found in dairy products. Complex carbohydrates are basically many simple sugars linked together. Complex carbohydrates are found in foods such as grains, pasta, rice, vegetables, breads, legumes, nuts, and seeds. Fiber is also considered a carbohydrate and is important to health; it is not, however, a nutrient, because most of it is not digested or absorbed into the body. Complex carbohydrates such as grains, vegetables, and legumes should supply the bulk of your carbohydrate calories since they supply a good bonus of vitamins, minerals, and fiber.

71. EAT MORE COMPLEX CARBOHYDRATES, LESS FAT AND PROTEIN

Healthy adults should consume approximately 55 percent of their total daily calories from carbohydrates. That means filling more than half of your plate with carbohydrate-rich foods such as grains, fruits, vegetables, and beans. The idea is to eat larger amounts of complex carbohydrates and smaller portions of protein and fat. Ounce for ounce, starches contain the same number of calories as protein and less than half the calories of fat. Carbohydrates and protein provide 4 calories per gram, and fat provides 9 calories per gram. To increase complex carbohydrates, use the following tips:

► Eat more fruits and vegetables.
► Eat more whole grains, rice, breads, and cereals.
► Eat more beans, lentils, and dried peas.

72. FOLLOW COMPLEX CARBOHYDRATE PROPORTION GUIDELINES

Health experts agree that you should consume at least half of your total daily calories from carbohydrates, especially complex carbohydrates. MyPyramid suggests consuming 5 to 8 ounces of grains per day depending on your age, sex, and level of physical activity. At least one-half of grains should be whole grains. Whole grain foods include:

► Brown rice
► Oatmeal
► Whole wheat bread
► Buckwheat
► Whole wheat pasta
► Popcorn

73. PACE YOURSELF

Your body converts all carbohydrates into glucose to be used as fuel or energy for the body. Glucose circulating in your bloodstream is known as blood sugar, which enters your body's cells, where it is converted to energy. Since simple carbohydrates, or simple sugars, are already in their simplest form, they go straight into the bloodstream. Complex carbohydrates require digestive enzymes to break them into glucose. Some glucose is used immediately for energy and some is stored in the liver and muscles in the form of glycogen. If you consume more calories than you need, excess glucose is also stored as fat. After you eat, the hormone insulin lowers the level of glucose in the blood by stimulating body cells to take up and store excess glucose. This helps to prevent your blood sugar from spiking too high. Another job of insulin is to help prevent too much glucose in the liver from being released between meals. At times when your blood sugar is low, such as after exercising or before breakfast, another hormone called glucagon stimulates the conversion of glycogen from the liver back to glucose for the body to use as energy. In simpler terms, insulin helps to regulate your blood sugar. By monitoring the rate and volume of complex carbs you consume, you can help your body function at high capacity and prevent it from adding fat cells.

74. EAT WHOLE GRAINS

Foods made from grains should be the base of a nutritious diet. Grains include bread, rice, pasta, and oats. Whole grain foods, especially whole grains, supply vitamin E and B vitamins such as folic acid as well as minerals like magnesium, iron, and zinc. Whole grains (like whole wheat) are rich in fiber and higher in other important nutrients. In fact, eating plenty of whole grain breads, bran cereals, and other whole-grain foods can easily provide half of your fiber needs for an entire day. When choosing grains, look for the words *whole grain* or *whole wheat* to make sure the product is made from 100 percent whole-wheat flour. The aim should be to consume at least six servings of grain products per day. Choose grains that are rich in fiber, low in saturated fat, and low in sodium.

75. LIMIT REFINED GRAINS

Refined grains include white bread and white rice. Whole grain is the entire edible part of any grain, including wheat, corn, oats, and rice. Refined grains go through a milling process in which parts of the grain are removed. In refined grains, many of the essential nutrients are lost in processing. Some nutrients are added back, or the product is enriched, but this usually does not include all of the nutrients that were lost. To make sure you eat more whole-grain foods rather than refined grains, look for words such as *whole grain, whole wheat, rye, bulgur, brown rice, oatmeal, whole oats, pearl barley,* and *whole-grain corn* as one of the first words in the ingredient list on a food label.

76. MAKE SMART STARCH CHOICES

MyPyramid suggests building a healthy base by making a variety of grain foods the foundation of your diet. To get the most out of this important food group, follow some of the following tips:

- ► Choose breads, cereals, and pastas made from whole wheat or whole grain more often. Rye and pumpernickel breads are also high in fiber.
- ► Look for the words *high in fiber* or *good source of fiber* on food labels.
- ► Look for breads, rolls, and muffins with 3 grams of fat or less per serving.
- ► Look for the word *whole* in front of grains such as barley, corn, oats, rice, or wheat.

- ▶ Choose brown rice more often than white. Brown rice is the only type of whole-grain rice.
- ▶ Look for varieties of cereal that offer at least 3 grams of fiber, have 3 grams of fat or less, and that include 8 grams or less of sugar per serving.

77. FOLLOW GRAIN PROPORTION GUIDELINES

One band of USDA's MyPyramid includes foods made from grains, and these foods should form the base of a nutritious diet. According to the USDA, consuming at least 3 or more ounce-equivalents of whole grains per day can reduce the risk of several chronic diseases and may help with weight maintenance. Thus, daily intake of at least 3 ounce-equivalents of whole grains per day is recommended by substituting whole grains for refined grains. At all calorie levels, all age groups should consume at least half the grains as whole grains to achieve the fiber recommendation. All grain servings can be whole-grain; however, it is advisable to include some folate-fortified products, such as folate-fortified whole-grain cereals, in these whole-grain choices.

78. EAT A VARIETY OF FRUITS AND VEGETABLES

Eating a variety of fruits and vegetables is key to a healthy diet. Fruits and vegetables are rich in different essential nutrients such as vitamins, minerals, and fiber. Eating a variety ensures a greater intake of these essential nutrients; aim to try different types and colors. Whether you are choosing fresh, frozen, canned, dried, or juice, you will receive the added benefits of this healthy food group. Juices and canned fruits do not provide as much fiber as the other types, so it is best to eat the fruit or vegetable more often. Eat at least five servings per day of fruits and vegetables, consisting of at least two servings of fruit and three servings of vegetables.

79. EAT NUTRIENT-RICH VEGETABLES

Vegetables are packed with all types of healthy nutrients. Daily requirements for several vitamins—including vitamin C, folic acid, and beta carotene, the precursor for vitamin A—can be met almost exclusively from fresh vegetables and fruits. This is especially true with dark-green leafy vegetables, such as spinach or broccoli, and dark orange vegetables, such as carrots or yams. Some vegetables also supply sufficient amounts of calcium, iron, and magnesium. In addition to nutrients, vegetables also contain phytochemicals that may provide additional health benefits. It's a good idea to load your diet with as many cruciferous vegetables as possible because of their cancer-preventing antioxidant properties (as well as other healthful benefits). The most potent cruciferous vegetables include bok choy (Chinese cabbage), broccoli, brussels sprouts, cabbage, cauliflower, collard greens, kale, mustard greens, rutabagas, turnips, and watercress. Also high in nutrition are carrots, celery, potatoes, spinach, sweet potatoes, and tomatoes (which contain a cancer-fighting compound known as lycopene).

80. FOLLOW VEGETABLE PROPORTION GUIDELINES

Vegetables are tasty and crunchy, and they can add lots of color and flavor to your meals. Vegetables are naturally low in calories. They have little to no fat, are cholesterol-free, and are packed with fiber. Eating a variety of colors and types ensures a better intake of all these nutrients. MyPyramid suggests consuming three to five servings from the vegetable group each day. One serving equals any of the following:

► ½ cup chopped raw, non-leafy vegetables
► ½ cup cooked vegetables
► ¾ cup vegetable juice

- ▸ 1 cup leafy, raw vegetables
- ▸ One small baked potato (3 ounces)
- ▸ ½ cup cooked legumes (beans, peas, or lentils)

81. EAT NUTRIENT-RICH FRUITS

Fruit's sweet flavor comes from fructose, a naturally occurring sugar that serves as a good source of energy. Fruit is full of healthy substances such as vitamin C, vitamin A, potassium, folic acid, antioxidants, phytochemicals, and fiber, just to name a few. Citrus fruits, berries, and melons are excellent sources of vitamin C. Dried fruits are available all year long and are an excellent source of many nutrients including fiber. Almost all fruits and vegetables are good for you, but some are better than others. When it comes to fruit, apples, bananas, berries, citrus fruit, and melons are your best bets because of their high fiber and nutrient content.

82. FOLLOW FRUIT PROPORTION GUIDELINES

The fruit and vegetable groups each have a band on the USDA's MyPyramid. Neither group is more important than the other, so you should eat servings from both groups. Most fruits have no fat, and all are cholesterol-free. Fruits are loaded with many essential nutrients that vary among the varieties. Eating different fruits ensures a better intake of all the nutrients that they provide. Try as many colors and types as you can for variety. MyPyramid suggests consuming two to four servings from the fruit group each day. One serving equals any of the following:

- ▸ One small to medium fresh fruit
- ▸ ½ cup canned or cut-up fresh fruit
- ▸ ¾ cup fruit juice
- ▸ ¼ cup dried fruit

83. OPT FOR 100 PERCENT FRUIT JUICE

When choosing fruit juices, check the label. Actual fruit juice contains fructose, the naturally occurring sugar in fruit. Fruit drinks, fruit cocktails, and fruitades contain fructose plus added sugar. When the label states "100 Percent Fruit Juice," the juice only has the naturally occurring fructose and no added sugar. The body uses all sugar the same, but juice with added sugar contains more calories. The percentage of juice has nothing to do with the nutrient content, such as vitamin C, so the best advice is to check out the food label.

84. CHOOSE LEAN PROTEIN

Protein is another macronutrient that is important to a healthy diet. Like carbohydrates, protein is made up of carbon, hydrogen, and oxygen. But proteins also contain nitrogen, which makes their role in the body's health unique. The body uses protein to build and repair bone, muscles, connective tissue, skin, internal organs, and blood. Protein also makes up your hair, nails, and teeth. Hormones, antibodies, and enzymes, which regulate the body's chemical reactions, are all composed of protein. Protein helps wounds to heal and blood to clot. If carbohydrates and fats can't meet your body's energy needs, protein can also be used as an energy source, because it provides calories. Protein can be found in meat, poultry, fish, eggs, milk, cheese, yogurt, and soy products. Legumes, seeds, and nuts also supply protein. Grain products and some vegetables supply smaller amounts of protein. Since Americans tend to use animal products to provide the majority of protein in their diet, and since animal products contain saturated fat and cholesterol, it is important to choose lower-fat dairy products and lean cuts of meat.

85. MEET YOUR AMINO ACID NEEDS

Protein is made up of building blocks called amino acids. There are about twenty different amino acids in the body that link in thousands of different ways to form thousands of different types of proteins. Each of these proteins has a unique function in the body. The amino acids must be arranged in a precise way to carry out their proper function. Deoxyribonucleic acid, or DNA, is the genetic code that carries instructions for the arrangement of each protein. Nine amino acids are classified as essential because your body does not make them and must get them from the foods you eat. Other amino acids are classified as nonessential because your body will make them if you consume enough essential amino acids and enough calories. Your body cannot directly use the protein you consume. Digestive enzymes break protein down into short amino-acid chains and then finally into individual amino acids. These amino acids can then enter the bloodstream and travel to the cells, where the body rebuilds them into the sequence or into the type of protein that it needs for a specific task. The body continually gets the amino acids it needs from a diet that meets your protein needs and from its own amino-acid pool. In general, animal proteins contain all nine of the essential amino acids and are therefore considered complete proteins. Foods such as legumes, vegetables, grains, nuts, and seeds are considered incomplete proteins because they are missing sufficient quantities of one or more essential amino acids.

86. KNOW YOUR RECOMMENDED DAILY PROTEIN

Protein needs are specific to your age and gender.

RECOMMENDED DAILY PROTEIN TABLE

Category	Age or Condition	Protein Grams
Males	15 to 18 years	59 grams
Males	19 to 24 years	58 grams
Males	25 to 50 years	63 grams
Males	51-plus years	63 grams
Females	11 to 14 years	46 grams
Females	15 to 18 years	44 grams
Females	19 to 24 years	46 grams
Females	25 to 50 years	50 grams
Females	51-plus years	50 grams
Pregnant		60 grams
Breastfeeding	First 6 months	65 grams
Breastfeeding	Second 6 months	62 grams

87. FAMILIARIZE YOURSELF WITH PROTEIN CONTENT

It is not hard to get your needed protein for the day. The numbers can add up quickly. Keep in mind the following protein contents of common foods:

- ▶ 1 cup of low-fat or fat-free milk contains 8 grams of protein.
- ▶ A 3- to 4-ounce serving of lean meat, poultry, or fish contains about 25 to 35 grams of protein. That is approximately the size of a deck of cards.
- ▶ 1 cup of cooked beans or lentils contains about 18 grams of protein.
- ▶ 1 cup of low-fat yogurt contains about 10 grams of protein.
- ▶ 1 cup of low-fat cottage cheese contains about 28 grams of protein.
- ▶ 2 tablespoons of peanut butter contains about 7 grams of protein.
- ▶ 2 ounces of low-fat cheese contains about 14 to 16 grams of protein.
- ▶ 1 egg contains about 7 grams of protein.
- ▶ 1 serving of vegetables contains around 1 to 3 grams of protein.
- ▶ 1 serving of grain foods generally contains 3 to 6 grams of protein.

88. FOLLOW MEAT (AND OTHER PROTEIN) PORTION GUIDELINES

Another band on the USDA's MyPyramid is the meat group. This group includes a variety of foods, including beef, pork, chicken, turkey, fish, game, eggs, dry beans (legumes, lentils, and peas), soy foods, nuts, and peanut butter. The meat group supplies large amounts of protein as well as other essential nutrients. Nuts, dry beans, and soy foods are grouped with meat because they are excellent sources of protein. You need fewer servings from the meat group because it is higher in fat. MyPyramid suggests consuming two to three servings or about 5 to 7 ounces from the meat group each day. One serving equals 2 to 3 ounces of cooked lean meat, poultry, or fish.

The following choices equal an ounce of meat:

- ► 1 egg
- ► ½ cup cooked legumes (lentils, peas, or dried beans)
- ► ¼ cup egg substitute
- ► 2 tablespoons peanut butter
- ► ⅓ cup nuts
- ► 4 ounces tofu
- ► 1 cup soy milk
- ► 2 to 3 ounces canned tuna or salmon, packed in water

89. EAT NUTRIENT-RICH, LEAN PROTEIN

Limit your consumption of red meat; the red meat you do eat should be as lean as possible. More healthful alternatives include poultry, legumes, and deep-water fish such as tuna, mackerel, herring, shrimp, and salmon, all of which contain nutritious omega-3 fatty acids.

90. MAKE HEALTHY PROTEIN CHOICES

The meat group is an important food group because of the nutrients it provides. However, because the majority of foods in the meat group contain saturated fat and cholesterol, it is important to make lean and low-fat choices. Follow these tips to help make low-fat choices from the meat group:

- ► When buying beef, be aware of grades and inspection of meat.
- ► Choose skinless, white meat poultry.
- ► Instead of ground beef, try lean ground turkey instead. Ground turkey breast can be up to 99 percent fat-free.

- ► Buy meat that is well trimmed, with no more than an eighth of an inch fat surrounding the cut of meat.
- ► When buying ground meats, look for packages that have the greatest percent lean-to-fat ratio.
- ► Choose beans, peas, lentils, and soy foods often, and try to make them your main meal several times per week.
- ► Limit your intake of high-fat processed meats, including bacon, sausage, bologna, salami, kielbasa, bratwurst, and other higher-fat meats.
- ► Limit your intake of liver and other organ meats that tend to be very high in cholesterol.
- ► Use egg yolks and whole eggs in moderation.
- ► Watch your portion sizes. Three ounces of cooked meat is about the size of a deck of cards.

91. MINIMIZE FAT THROUGH COOKING METHODS

With a few simple tips, you can make a big difference in reducing total fat, saturated fat, and cholesterol in your meals. Try the following techniques:

- ► Trim all visible fat from meat before cooking.
- ► Use low-fat cooking methods: broil, grill, roast, braise, stew, steam, poach, stir-fry, or microwave.
- ► Brown meat in a nonstick skillet with little to no fat. Use a vegetable oil spray to prevent sticking.
- ► When grilling, broiling, or roasting meat and poultry, use a rack for the fat to drip through.
- ► Use marinades for meat that have little to no fat: light teriyaki sauce, orange juice, lime juice, lemon juice, tomato juice, defatted broth, or low-fat yogurt.

Add fresh herbs and other spices such as garlic powder to marinades for more flavor.

▶ Oven bake fish and chicken instead of frying.

92. DON'T GO OVERBOARD

When it comes to protein, the body uses only what it needs. Extra protein is not stored in the body as protein for future use; it's either used as energy or stored as body fat. Eating large amounts of protein, especially from animal foods, can increase your saturated fat (bad fat) and cholesterol intake. It can also cause nutrient imbalances by crowding out other important foods such as grains, fruits, and vegetables and put an extra strain on the kidneys. When protein is digested, it produces toxic by-products, and it is the kidney's job to filter them out. Also, consumption of excess protein requires more water to excrete the urea, a waste product formed when protein turns to body fat. This increases the chances for dehydration and increases the need to urinate.

93. DON'T BULK UP TO BUILD MUSCLES

The only thing that builds bigger muscles is exercise and working your muscles. Consuming extra amounts of protein from either food or supplements really has no added benefit. Athletes only need slightly more protein than the RDAs. Generally, nonathletes need around ½ gram per pound of body weight and most athletes need ½ to ¾ grams of protein per pound of body weight.

94. ALWAYS INCLUDE DAIRY

The milk group is another band on the USDA's MyPyramid, next to but larger than the meat group. The milk group includes milk and foods made from milk, such as yogurt, cheese, cottage cheese, buttermilk, frozen yogurt, and ice cream. The milk group, especially milk, yogurt, and cheese, is an excellent source of calcium and riboflavin, and provides many essential vitamins and minerals, as well as protein. According to the National Dairy Council, "Intake of fluid milk has been demonstrated to reduce the risk of osteoporosis, hypertension, and colon cancer. Drinking milk may help to reduce the risk of kidney stones. Milk intake may help to reduce the risk of tooth decay by acting as a substitute for saliva." Dairy foods are good sources of protein, calcium, riboflavin, phosphorus, potassium, vitamin A, and vitamin D. The dairy group is one of the biggest contributors to calcium intake, which is extremely important for bone health.

95. OPT FOR SKIM

Dairy foods, unfortunately, are also a source of fat and cholesterol. Since dairy products are animal products, the majority of the fat they contain is saturated (the bad fat). Choosing lower-fat and fat-free versions can decrease fat and cholesterol intake. Skim milk has all the important nutrients in the same quantity as low-fat or whole milk.

96. FOLLOW DAIRY PROPORTION GUIDELINES

Fewer servings are needed from the milk group compared to other food groups because dairy foods are naturally higher in fat. Smaller amounts from the milk group will still provide the nutrients that you need. MyPyramid suggests consuming two to three servings from the milk group each day. One serving equals any of the following:

- ▶ 1 cup low-fat or fat-free milk
- ▶ 2 ounces processed cheese
- ▶ 1 cup low-fat yogurt

- ⅓ cup dry milk
- 1½ ounces natural cheese
- ¾ cup low-fat cottage cheese

97. TRY LACTOSE-FREE

Dairy foods contain a natural occurring sugar called lactose. During digestion of dairy foods, an enzyme called lactase breaks down lactose to make it easily digestible. People who are lactose-intolerant produce too little of this enzyme. Left undigested, lactose can cause nausea, cramping, bloating, gas, and diarrhea. Some people are more tolerant than others and can eat dairy products in different amounts. If you are lactose-intolerant, choose low-lactose or lactose-free dairy products. A majority of lactose-intolerant people can eat yogurt with no symptoms.

98. EMBRACE (GOOD) FAT

Fat is another macronutrient vital to a healthy diet. In fact, fat is a very con-centrated source of energy, providing more than double the amount of calories in one gram of carbohydrate or protein. Fats are made up of carbon, hydrogen, and oxygen molecules. The general term for fat found in food is *triglyceride*. We need moderate amounts of fat in our diets to perform important functions. Fat helps carry, absorb, and store the fat-soluble vitamins (A, D, E, and K) in your bloodstream. Without fat, these vitamins would not be able to nourish the body. A certain amount of body fat is needed to cushion your organs and protect them from injury and to supply insulation to help regulate body temperature.

99. FOLLOW FAT PROPORTION GUIDELINES

Health experts agree that you should get no more than 30 percent of your total calories from fat. They also recommend consuming no more than 10 percent of that 30 percent from saturated sources of fat and no more than 7 percent if you have coronary heart disease, diabetes, or high-LDL cholesterol. Eating any type of fat in excess can cause weight gain because it is higher in calories. Overloading on specific types of fat, such as saturated fat, can also put you at risk for serious health problems.

100. MINIMIZE FATS AND OILS,

Fats and oils, although not a food group, are included in MyPyramid. These foods include foods that are mostly fat or sugar, such as oils, salad dressings, cream, butter, gravy, margarine and cream cheese. These foods supply calories but little in the way of nutrients. Since fats and oils are not considered a food group, they have no recommended serving ranges, etc.

101. WATCH FAT CONSUMPTION

Dietary fats and oils, or triglycerides, are a source of energy and help produce compounds that regulate a variety of bodily functions, including blood clotting and blood pressure. They can be saturated or unsaturated, and unsaturated fats can be either monounsaturated or polyunsaturated. All triglycerides supply approximately 250 calories per ounce—more than double the calories supplied by equal amounts of protein or carbohydrates. Keep your fat consumption on the low side.

102. CHOOSE GOOD FATS

Over half of our brain matter consists of fats or lipids that create all the cell membranes in the body. If you eat bad fats, you make low-quality nerve cell membranes; if you eat good fats, you make higher-quality nerve cell membranes and influence positively the action of nerve cells. Certain foods containing omega-3 fatty acids, such as certain cold-water fish, olive oil, flaxseed oil, peanut oil, canola oil, and certain fish oils have the real potential to help the brain. A 2003 study organized by the Rush-Presbyterian-St. Luke's Medical Center in Chicago found that those who ate fish at least once a week had a 60 percent less chance of developing Alzheimer's than those who rarely ate fish. Fish that provide omega-3 oils include: bluefish, herring, mackerel, rainbow trout, salmon, sardines, tuna, and whitefish.

103. LIMIT SATURATED AND HYDROGENATED FATS

The most important nutrients in the brain are essential fatty acids; our diet, however, is sorely lacking in the essential fats from flaxseed oil, olive oil, and fish oil, but is overabundant in saturated, hydrogenated, and partially hydrogenated trans fats found in all commercial baked goods, margarines, and processed foods. Saturated fats tend to raise cholesterol levels and thus endanger your heart and your brain. Saturated fats are usually solid at room temperature and can be found in well-marbled meat, butter, whole milk cheese, ice cream, egg yolks, and fatty cuts of beef, pork, and lamb. Certain vegetable oils, such as palm, palm kernel, and coconut oils are also saturated. According to the APF's Alzheimer's Prevention Program, the first dietary recommendation is to reduce fat intake to about 15 to 20 percent of your total calories. But they also say that even more important is the quality of the fats that you eat. Stay away from these bad boys.

104. BAN TRANS FATS

Trans fats are artificially produced solid fats created by heating liquid vegetable oils in the presence of metal catalysts and hydrogen. This process, called partial hydrogenation, causes carbon atoms to bond in a straight configuration and remain solid at room temperature. Naturally occurring unsaturated fatty acids have carbon atoms that line up in a bent shape, resulting in a liquid state at room

temperature. Trans fats may be even more harmful than saturated and hydrogenated fats. They disrupt the production of energy in the mitochondria (the energy
factories) of brain cells. When it comes to trans fats, just say no.

105. MAKE DAILY LOW-FAT CHOICES

It is important to include fat in your daily diet but in moderation. Eating a completely fat-free diet is *not* part of a healthy eating style. To help you incorporate
fat in moderation in your diet, use some of the following tips:

▶ Choose low-fat or fat-free dairy products.
▶ Use low-fat dressings and limit buttermilk, ranch, or blue cheese dressings.
▶ Use nonstick cooking sprays or nonstick pans and avoid frying anything in oil.
▶ Trim excess fat and skin from all meat and poultry.
▶ Choose based on amount of total fat and type of fat.
▶ Watch for hidden fats: pizza toppings, fried foods, ice cream, high-fat meats
  (salami, bologna, bratwurst, hot dogs, pepperoni, sausage, bacon, and spare
  ribs), cakes, cookies, macaroni salad, potato salad, and coleslaw.
▶ Limit your intake of red meat; opt for poultry, fish, or nonmeat dishes more often.
▶ Limit pastas in cream sauces; use marinara or other tomato-based
  toppings instead. ✳

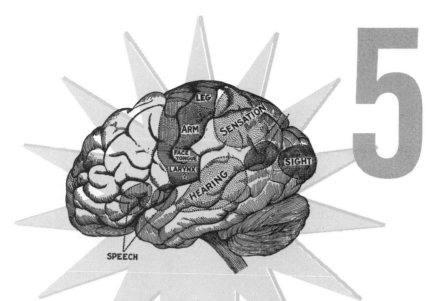

5

FEED YOUR BRAIN—SUPERFOODS

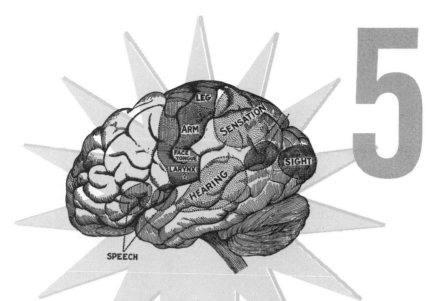

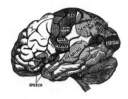

FEED YOUR BRAIN— SUPERFOODS

When it comes to brain protection, there's nothing quite like blueberries.

106. PICK THE SUPERFOODS

Some foods are better for you than others. The key is to eat a diverse diet, with an emphasis on those foods with nutritional punch. The majority of Americans don't consume nearly enough fruits and vegetables. Government health officials suggest five servings of fruit and vegetables daily—twice the amount suggested for meat and dairy. Fruits and vegetables are an important part of any anti-aging regimen because they are packed with essential nutrients in their most natural and useful form.

107. DRINK GREEN TEA

The research on green tea and green tea extract is extensive—and impressive. Here are some findings thus far:

► Countries that have a high consumption of green tea had lower rates of cancer.
► Green tea can block the development of angiogenesis—the new blood vessels needed by tumors in order for their cells to colonize and grow. Animal studies

showed that the consumption of two or three cups of green tea daily was sufficient to significantly suppress tumor growth.

▶ Smokers who drink green tea—only about three cups daily—had less occurrence of lung damage than those who do not.

▶ Green tea extract can inhibit bacteria that cause periodontal disease and cavities; as a mouth rinse, it can reduce plaque.

▶ Women over the age of forty who were not cigarette smokers and who drank five or more cups of green tea daily had half the incidence of stroke as those who drank less.

▶ Green tea contains catechins, which inhibit the proliferation of smooth muscle cells lining blood vessels, a process that can help prevent atherosclerosis and heart disease.

▶ The consumption of ten cups of green tea (or more) daily can protect against liver damage (from alcohol and other toxins).

A healthy heart means healthy circulation and that benefits your brain enormously. Drink up!

108. EAT YOUR OATMEAL

Studies have shown that foods such as oatmeal that are high in soluble fiber may help to lower LDL cholesterol without lowering HDL cholesterol. Whether you choose steel-cut oats (the most roughly cut and least processed), rolled or "old-fashioned" oats, quick oats, or instant, all types of oats are effective at reducing cholesterol. To get the daily 3 grams of soluble fiber recommended for cholesterol lowering, you'll need to eat: 2 ounces of oat bran (⅔ cup dry or about 1½ cups cooked) or 3 ounces of oatmeal (1 cup dry or 2 cups cooked).

109. EAT MORE WILD SALMON

The omega-3 fatty acids present in salmon puts this fish at the top of the super-foods chart. Salmon provides two types of omega-3s: DHA (docosahexaenoic acid) and EPA (eicosapentaenoic acid); and it's high in vitamin D, selenium, protein, and B vitamins. Some studies have found that omega-3s can significantly decrease serum triglyceride levels, lower blood pressure, and reduce blood levels of homocysteine, high levels of which are associated with an increased risk of heart disease, stroke, Alzheimer's disease, Parkinson's disease, and osteoporosis. Omega-3s also help to thin the blood by discouraging platelets in the blood from clumping together, thus reducing the risk that the blood will clot and cause a heart attack. Preliminary research also suggests that omega-3 fatty acids from fish oil may help regulate the rhythm of the heart, as both EPA and DHA have been reported to help prevent cardiac arrhythmias. Potent anti-inflammatory agents, omega-3s help curb an overactive immune system and thus are helpful in the treatment of autoimmune diseases such as rheumatoid arthritis, chronic inflammatory bowel disease, Crohn's disease, and psoriasis. Wild salmon has more nutrients and fewer pollutants than farm-raised salmon so opt for it as often as possible.

110. EAT MORE SOY

According to experts, soy protein appears to help prevent heart disease by lowering blood cholesterol levels; decreasing blood clots and platelet "clumping" or aggregation (both of which can increase the risk for a heart attack or stroke); improving the elasticity of arteries (which makes blood flow better); and reducing oxidation of low-density lipoprotein (LDL or "bad" cholesterol), which can lower the risk of plaque formation. The Food and Drug Administration is so convinced of soy's benefits that the agency approved a health claim for soy protein and heart disease in October 1999. Good sources include defattened soy flour, isolated soy protein, miso, firm tofu, soy cheese, regular tofu, soymilk, and soy veggie burgers. Adding one serving a day can make a difference. Soy up!

111. EAT KALE AND OTHER BRASSICA VEGETABLES

Loaded with cancer-fighting antioxidants, kale is, literally, one of the healthiest foods in the vegetable kingdom. Together with its cousin, broccoli, kale offers strong protection against cancer and other disease. Kale and other Brassica vegetables contain a potent glucosinolate phytonutrient, which actually boosts your body's detoxification enzymes clearing potentially carcinogenic substances more quickly from your body. More common members of the prestigious Brassica family of vegetables include: cabbage, broccoli, brussels sprouts, cauliflower, kale, collards, mustard greens, rapini, bok choy, and broccoli rabe. With so many choices take advantage of having one variety each day of the week.

112. EAT AN APPLE

Studies have shown that apples may be instrumental as a preventative for heart disease, some types of stroke, and even cancer. The active ingredient in apple pulp is pectin, a soluble form of fiber that helps reduce "bad" cholesterol by keeping it in the intestinal tract until it is eliminated. A study published in the *Journal of the National Cancer Institute* shows that pectin binds certain cancer-causing compounds in the colon, accelerating their removal from the body. European studies indicate that apple pectin can help to eliminate lead, mercury, and other toxic heavy metals from the human body. Note: It's important to thoroughly wash apples and to avoid eating the seeds, which can be poisonous. All apples provide super nutrients, but eating a variety of apples is even better.

113. EAT A NUT

Nuts are high in fat but they contain minerals, fiber, and nice amounts of protein. All nuts and seeds are small powerhouses in themselves. So powerful, in fact, that just having a serving of nuts five times a week can significantly reduce your risk for heart disease. Nuts are high in calories so should be eaten in moderation; think of a serving as a tablespoon or two. Look for nuts that are unsalted; it's not important whether they are roasted or unroasted. Nuts are great sprinkled on foods high in vitamin C, such as fruit and vegetables, because the vitamin C increases the body's absorption of the iron in nuts.

114. EAT WALNUTS IN PARTICULAR

If for no other reason, the walnut is the only nut that provides significant amounts of alpha-linolenic acid, one of the three omega-3 fatty acids. Because your body cannot produce this acid it needs to be provided daily from other sources. All it takes is seven walnuts to supply your daily need for these essential fatty acids. Omega-3s are your brain food, and the high amounts of unsaturated fat help to lower the LDL or "bad" cholesterol in your blood and increase HDL, the "good" cholesterol. By eating a handful of walnuts a day you can reduce your risk for heart disease.

115. MUNCH ON PUMPKIN SEEDS

Pumpkin seeds, also known as pepitas, nestle in the core of the pumpkin encased in a white-yellow husk. This super seed contains a number of minerals, such as zinc, magnesium, manganese, iron, copper, phosphorus, along with proteins, monounsaturated fat, and the omega fatty acids 3 and 6. Today the super powers of pumpkin seeds have been found to help prevent prostate cancer in men, protect against heart disease, and also have anti-inflammatory benefits.

116. EAT AN EGG

Once the victim of a bad rap, nutritional research has shown that an egg has protein (in the white part) and fat (in the yellow part), but no carbohydrates. The white has few other nutrients, while the yellow has a high amount of vitamin B_{12} and folate. Nutritionists used to think that eggs contained too much fat, but now they know that the fat in an egg is good for the brain and doesn't contribute to higher levels of cholesterol in the blood. Bad news for chickens; good news for your brain.

117. EAT A SWEET POTATO

Sweet potatoes have high amounts of beta carotene, equal to that of carrots; and for 90 calories per sweet potato you get a huge amount of health-building nutrients. Beta carotene is a major fighter against cancer, heart disease, asthma, and rheumatoid arthritis. The bright orange flesh of the sweet potato contains carotenoids that help stabilize your blood sugar and lower insulin resistance, making cells more responsive to insulin, and aiding your metabolism. Sweet potatoes have four times the USRDA for beta carotene when eaten with the skin on. In fact, it would take twenty cups of broccoli to provide the 38,000 IUs of beta carotene (vitamin A) available in one cup of cooked sweet potatoes. They are a source of vitamin E, vitamin B_6, potassium, and iron, plus they're fat-free. Cup for cup, sweet potatoes have been found to provide as much fiber as oatmeal.

118. EAT CEREAL

Cereal grains should also be a big part of your daily diet. They provide much-needed fiber as well as a variety of important vitamins and minerals. Obviously, this refers to low-fat, low-sugar cereals, such as natural granola, oatmeal, bran, bran flakes, etc. Fortified cereals offer another source of vitamins.

119. EAT BROCCOLI SPROUTS

Researchers estimate that broccoli sprouts provide 10 to 100 times the power of mature broccoli to neutralize carcinogens. Dr. Talalay, MD, researcher at the Johns Hopkins School of Medicine, found that three-day-old broccoli sprouts consistently contained twenty to fifty times the amount of chemo-protective compounds found in mature broccoli heads, thereby offering a simple, dietary means of chemically reducing cancer risk. These super sprouts boost enzymes in the body, while detoxifying potential carcinogens. The antioxidants found in broccoli sprouts may help prevent several types of cancer, heart disease, macular degeneration, and stomach ulcer and may also help reduce cholesterol levels.

120. EAT BLUEBERRIES

In a *Newsweek* article dated June 17, 2002, neuroscientist James Joseph of Tufts University made it clear that when it comes to brain protection, there's nothing quite like blueberries, which he calls the "brain berry." Dr. Joseph attributes its health benefits to antioxidant and anti-inflammatory compounds and sees its potential for reversing short-term memory loss and forestalling many other effects of aging. In a study on reversing memory loss reported in the *Wall Street Journal*, blueberries had the strongest impact on the mental function of aging rodents than any of the other fruits tested. The American Institute for Cancer Research recommends eating blueberries because they are "one of the best sources of antioxidants, substances that can slow the aging process and reduce cell damage that can lead to cancer." By eating only half a cup of fresh or frozen blueberries a day you can receive their antioxidant protection and benefit from their anti-aging properties. When out of season buy them frozen to have in a smoothie or mixed with yogurt and walnuts as a delicious snack.

121. REPLACE RED WINE WITH A BLUEBERRY SMOOTHIE

A report published in the *Journal of Agriculture and Food Chemistry* showed that the blueberry has 38 percent more antioxidants than red wine. One cup of blueberries reportedly provides three to five times the antioxidants found in five servings of carrots, broccoli, squash, and apples. What this means for your health is a lower risk of heart disease; vibrant, firm skin; and a boost in brain power.

122. PILE ON THE GARLIC

Garlic lowers cholesterol levels, thins the blood, kills bacteria, boosts the immune system, lowers blood sugar levels, and reduces risk of certain types of cancer. It may also help relieve asthma, ease ear infections, and facilitate healthy cell function. Incorporate fresh garlic into salads by chopping, crushing, or putting through a garlic press (2 or 3 cloves a day is optimum). Whole garlic bulbs can be roasted in the oven and the individual cloves squeezed out onto bread or toast as a creamy spread. Capsules: Take 1 to 3 capsules daily, or follow the label directions. While more may be best, some is definitely good for your circulatory system, and thus your brain.

123. EAT QUINOA

Once known as "the gold of the Incas," this complete protein includes all nine essential amino acids, which makes it an excellent choice for vegetarians, vegans, and the rest of the population. Quinoa has extra-high amounts of the amino acid lysine, which is essential for tissue growth and repair. It is also a very good source of manganese as well as magnesium, iron, copper, phosphorus, and the B-vitamins, especially folate, another essential nutrient needed for the formation and development of new and normal body tissue (one your body must acquire from foods and supplements). The other B vitamin quinoa provides is riboflavin or B_2, which is necessary for the proper production of cellular energy in your body. By improving the energy metabolism within the brain and muscle cells, B2 may help reduce the frequency of migraine attacks. Combine this protein with quinoa's high amounts of potassium and magnesium content to help lower your blood pressure and strengthen your heart. For such a small "grain," quinoa not only provides a whole lot of nutrients, but also may be especially valuable for persons with migraine headaches, diabetes, atherosclerosis, and other debilitating health issues.

124. EAT SEA VEGETABLES

Gram for gram, sea vegetables are higher in essential vitamins and minerals than any other known food group. These minerals are bio-available to the body in chelated, colloidal forms that make them more easily absorbed. Sea vegetables that provide minerals in this colloidal form have been shown to retain their molecular identity while remaining in liquid suspension. The following is a descriptive list of what sea vegetables can add to your daily diet:

▶ Sea vegetables can contain as much as 48 percent protein.
▶ Sea vegetables are a rich source of both soluble and insoluble dietary fiber.
▶ The brown sea vegetable varieties—kelp, wakame, and kombu—contain alginic acid, which has been shown to remove heavy metals and radioactive isotopes from the digestive tract.
▶ Sea vegetables contain significant amounts of vitamin A, in the form of beta carotene, as well as vitamins B complex, C, and E.
▶ Sea vegetables are high in potassium, calcium, sodium, iron, and chloride.
▶ Sea vegetables provide the fifty-six minerals and trace minerals that your body requires to function properly.

Today sea vegetables are available from the Maine Coast Sea Vegetable Company on the east coast and the Mendocino Sea Vegetable Company in northern California.

125. CONSUME MICRO-PLANTS

Micro-plants consisting of blue-green algae, chlorella, spirulina, wheat grass, and barley grass contain more vitamins and minerals than kale and broccoli. They are an excellent source of two important phytochemicals: chlorophyll and lycopene. Micro-plants, commercially known as *green foods*, contain a concentrated combination of phytochemicals, vitamins, minerals, bioflavanoids, proteins, amino acids, essential fatty acids, enzymes, coenzymes, and fiber. They support your body's ability to detoxify heavy metals, pesticides, and other toxins, plus boost your immunity to disease. Dr. Richard Schulze, author of *Get Well*, refers to micro-plants as nature's blood transfusion.

126. THROW IN SOME PARSLEY

Parsley is loaded with compounds that purify your blood and expel toxins from your body. It is also dense in vitamin C, vitamin A, vitamin K, iodine, iron, and chlorophyll. Actually, parsley has a higher vitamin C content than citrus, and thus is an excellent ingredient to battle inflammation. It also contains certain volatile oils that have been shown to inhibit the formation of tumors, particularly in the lungs. Parsley is also rich in flavonoids known for their antioxidant activity and helps to prevent free radical damage to your body's cells. Parsley's dark green color provides needed oxygenating chlorophyll increasing the antioxidant capacity of your blood. The body parts most affected by the properties in parsley are the kidneys, bladder, stomach, liver, and gall bladder.

127. CHOMP ON CHIVES

Chives and chive flowers are high in vitamin C, folic acid, potassium, calcium, and blood-building iron; and they stimulate the appetite and promote good digestion, reduce flatulence, and prevent bad breath. Chives, when eaten regularly, may help to lower blood cholesterol levels. Because of their high vitamin C content, they can help prevent colds or speed recovery from a cold; the sulfurous compounds in them are natural expectorants. Best used fresh, they are easy to grow in pots at home.

128. CURRY FAVOR

Turmeric (*Curcuma longa*), a common ingredient in curry powder, has a beneficial effect on digestion; it stimulates the flow of bile and the breakdown of dietary fats. German research indicates that turmeric can protect against gall-bladder disorders and is an effective treatment for gall-bladder disease. But more importantly, according to Earl Mindell's *Herb Bible*, "The herbs that are combined to make curry help prevent heart disease and stroke by reducing cholesterol and preventing clots."

129. SPICE IT UP

The red hot chili known as cayenne is used today as a potent stimulant for the whole body and considered a tonic for the nervous system. Hot herbs are supposed to increase metabolism rate and cayenne may help with weight loss. Recently, research has suggested that cayenne can ease the severe pain of shingles and migraines. It is readily available in powered form or as a bottled hot sauce.

130. EAT AVOCADOS

Avocados contain monounsaturated fat known as oleic acid, which has been shown to help lower cholesterol, prevent heart disease and arteriosclerosis, and lower your risk for cancer. They are also magnesium-rich, as well as loaded with potassium, which helps to regulate blood pressure and prevent circulatory diseases, including high blood pressure, stroke, and heart disease. One cup of avocado contains 23 percent of the daily value for folate, which when combined with the monounsaturated fats plus potassium, decreases your chances of cardio-vascular disease and stroke. Ounce for ounce, avocados provide more magnesium than the twenty most commonly eaten fruits. They contain no starch and very little sugar, yet they provide an excellent source of usable food energy. However, one whole California avocado has over 300 calories and 35 grams of fat, 8.5 grams being monounsaturated fat, so eat small amounts for the optimum benefit.

131. EAT CHOCOLATE FOR YOUR BRAIN

In a study done by Salk Institute researcher Henriette van Praag and colleagues, a compound found in cocoa, epicatechin, combined with exercise, was found to promote functional changes in a part of the brain involved in the formation of learning and memory. Epicatechin is one of a group of chemicals called flavo-nols, which have previously been shown to improve cardiovascular function and increase blood flow to the brain. Dr. van Praag's findings, published in the May 30, 2007 issue of *The Journal of Neuroscience*, suggest a diet rich in flavonoids could help reduce the effects of neurodegenerative illnesses such as Alzheimer's disease or cognitive disorders related to aging.

132. EAT CHOCOLATE FOR YOUR HEART

Dark chocolate may help lower blood pressure in people with hypertension, and has been shown to decrease levels of LDL, the "bad" cholesterol, by 10 percent. Including dark chocolate in your diet may benefit your heart by helping to block arterial damage caused by free radicals; and inhibit platelet aggregation, which could cause a heart attack or stroke. There have also been studies indicating that the flavonoids in cocoa relax the blood vessels, which inhibits an enzyme that causes inflammation.

133. OPT FOR DARK CHOCOLATE

According to study results published in the American Chemical Society's *Journal of Agriculture and Food Chemistry*, cocoa powder has nearly twice the antioxidants in red wine and up to three times what is found in green tea. Based on the U.S. Department of Agriculture / American Chemical Society's findings, dark chocolate tested the highest for antioxidants over other fruits and vegetables. Comparing the levels of antioxidants dark chocolate came in with a score of 13,120; Its closest competitor milk chocolate had levels of 6,740 and third was prunes at 5,770.

134. BUY QUALITY CHOCOLATES

Inexpensive chocolates are often blended with wax, and contain very little real cocoa butter. Inexpensive brands are also made with partially hydrogenated palm oil, preservatives, and high amounts of sugar. Quality chocolate is made using real cocoa butter, the finest organic cocoa beans, minimal sugar, and an extensive refining process. To counter the sugar, saturated fats, and artificial flavorings in commercial candy bars, many people have turned to buying chocolate in its raw, organic form and making their own sweets.

135. MUNCH ON OLIVES

Olives, long an essential part of the Mediterranean diet, are delicious, and their oil, high in monounsaturated fats, has recently hit the headlines because of its ability to reduce "bad" cholesterol in the blood. Dr. Andrew Weil recommends the exclusive use of olive oil for fat in the diet. Studies have shown that people who consume olive oil in preference to other fats have a lower incidence of heart disease. ✳

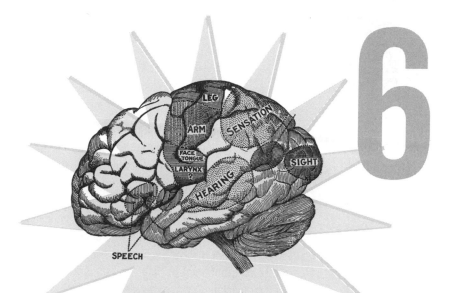

SUPPLEMENT YOUR BRAIN WITH HERBS

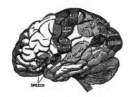

6

SUPPLEMENT YOUR BRAIN WITH HERBS

Herbs can relieve stress, improve circulations, and even boost memory.

136. CONSIDER HERBS

Recent studies show that more than 75 percent of Americans now use some form of alternative healing for their health care with the result that herbal remedies have become immensely popular as natural health promoters, and as complements to over-the-counter drugstore medicines as well as prescription drugs. Even the American academic establishment is getting into the herbal medicine act, with major U.S. research centers now investigating the healing potential of herbs and other alternative medical approaches. Always consult with your physician before ingesting herbal remedies, particularly if you are pregnant.

137. EMBRACE HERBS

Modern science and technology are studying the burgeoning herbal pharmacopoeia. Researchers are finding that wild plants contain a storehouse of genetic information that may lead to new treatments for disease, especially those that have heretofore resisted treatment, such as AIDS and other immune-deficiency diseases. Keep an open mind when it comes to herbs and their potent benefits. Your brain will thank you later.

138. CONSIDER THE DIFFERENCES BETWEEN HERBAL REMEDIES AND DRUGS

There are some vital differences between herbal remedies and drugs.

Herbal Medicines	Conventional Drugs
Are based on entire, whole plant	Are based on isolated chemicals
Are made from natural substances	May be synthetic
Are created from the sun's energy	Are unrelated to Nature's cycle
Have few if any side effects	Always have side effects
Work slowly and subtly	Work dramatically
Enhance vitality	Deplete vitality

139. RESEARCH HERBS

In recent years, innumerable books on herbs, herbal medicine, herbal remedies, and herbal preparations of all kinds have rolled off the printing presses. The shelves of both libraries and bookstores are lined with them. Here are two resources that will offer information.

- You can "Ask Dr. Weil" at *www.drweil.com.* Andrew Weil, MD, has archived according to date all of his findings, which guarantees the latest research information.
- Just about everything you'd want to know about 2,500 herbs and their properties can be found in *The Herb Book* by John Lust, which many nutritionists consider the most complete catalog of nature's miracle plants ever published.

140. SEE IT FROM A DOCTOR'S VIEWPOINT

If you are interested in having a doctor's opinion on any herbal remedies you would like to investigate or to take, there is a book available, by Volker Schultz, Rudolf Hansel, and Varro E. Tyler, PhD, ScD, that was written especially for physicians titled *Rational Phytotherapy: A Physicians' Guide to Herbal Medicine.*

141. LEARN THE FACTS

If you want to see for yourself what the current state of scientific research is on herbs and other supplements, you can visit the new database *(http://ods.od.nih .gov/Health_Information/IBIDS.aspx)* created by the Office of Dietary Supplements at the National Institutes of Health, which maintains a list of credible scientific studies on herbs, and everything else that is classified as "dietary supplements." Called IBIDS (International Bibliographic Information on Dietary Supplements), the site permits you to search at no charge on hundreds of topics—just name your herb. With one mouse click, IBIDS will research your chosen herb in medical, botanical, and pharmaceutical databases, and display a list of relevant studies.

You can save study titles and summaries and send them to your e-mail account. The site also offers links to over a thousand medical and scientific journals that provide you with the entire text of any study you choose.

142. ALWAYS CONSULT YOUR DOCTOR FIRST

Don't ever self-prescribe without a professional diagnosis. Even healthy adults should always consult their physician before taking herbs for medicinal purposes. When using herbs to treat any specific ailment for which you are also consulting a medical doctor, be sure to advise your doctor. Never discontinue conventional treatment or use any herbs in conjunction with it without the approval of your medical advisor. **Caution**: Although many herbs can safely be given to children, always check with a qualified pediatrician before administering herbal remedies to a child. Ditto for pregnant women—never take herbal preparations without consulting your obstetrician.

143. CONSULT A NATUROPATH

Medical professionals specially trained in natural medicine, called naturopaths, are fully licensed MD's who generally recommend natural approaches for the treatment of health problems. To find a naturopath in your area, contact the American Association of Naturopathic Physicians, 601 Valley Street, Suite 105, Seattle, WA 98109 (206-298-0125 or *www.naturopathic.org*). Naturopathic doctors' fees vary anywhere from $35 to $175 for an initial consultation, but you can expect the naturopathic practitioner to spend considerably more time with you than does the average MD, especially those who work for HMOs. And naturopathic doctors typically offer the same level of professionalism as does a regular MD.

144. BUY QUALITY PRODUCTS

When buying packaged herbal products, choose a reliable brand and follow the manufacturer's directions concerning dosage. Buy only from reputable manufacturers. The label should include the company's address, batch and lot numbers, expiration date, and recommended dosage.

145. USE AS DIRECTED

Of the herbs mentioned here, most are considered reasonably safe when recommendations for usage are followed. Such directions may vary from manufacturer to manufacturer due to factors such as potency, so always read the labels and follow their explicit instructions. As with any substance, excess can do harm, but there is little harm to be found with herbs when they are administered properly. Discuss any concerns with your doctor, not the health food store clerk.

146. WATCH FOR SIDE EFFECTS

If you experience *any* side effects, discontinue use at once and consult your physician. You can also call the FDA hot line at 800-322-1088 to report adverse side effects or online at *www.fda.gov/medwatch/how.htm*. For information about the safe use of botanicals, visit the American Botanical Council's website at *abc.herbalgram.org*.

147. BE AWARE OF BLOOD PRESSURE CAUTIONS

People taking medication to lower their blood pressure should avoid licorice (the herb, not the candy), mistletoe, and eleuthero, according to Varro E. Tyler, PhD, ScD, advisor to *Prevention* magazine. Tyler also warns those using thyroid medication to avoid bugleweed, which can further decrease thyroid activity.

148. TAKE ALFALFA

Modern-day scientists have discovered that alfalfa can be an agent in the treatment of heart disease, stroke, and cancer—the top three causes of death in the United States. Its leaves—which contain its real healing properties—are rich in minerals and other nutrients, including calcium, magnesium, potassium, and beta carotene, and may reduce "bad" cholesterol. Alfalfa leaf is on the FDA's list of herbs generally regarded as safe, but it should be used in medicinal amounts only with your doctor's approval. If you experience any side effects—such as upset stomach or diarrhea—stop use. **Caution:** Alfalfa seeds are to be avoided entirely, especially by anyone with an autoimmune problem.

149. TAKE PRIMROSE CAPSULES

Evening primrose oil is high in linoleic acid and has been shown to help lower blood cholesterol, which is good for your circulatory system, and thus good for your brain. The usual dose is one 250 milligram capsule three times a day. Swedish studies, though preliminary, are relating evening primrose oil to an antioxidant that counteracts the formation of free radicals, which are especially active in the aging process.

150. TAKE GINKGO BILOBA

The leaves of the ginkgo contain the active constituents ginkgo flavone glycosides and terpene lactones, the extract of which can be used to treat poor circulation in the legs as well as memory and cognitive problems. In a study published in the *Journal of the American Medical Association* researchers confirmed that people who take the ginkgo extract for mild to severe dementia may improve both their ability to remember and to interact socially. Usual dosage for extract: 120 to 240 milligrams daily, in 3 doses. Plan to take it for at least eight weeks before improvement shows. For capsules: Depending on capsule strength of the product you buy, use the same amount as the above recommended dosage. The standard dose is 40 to 60 milligrams. Buy a quality product and read the label. Look for products marked "24/6," an indication the product contains 24 percent flavone glycosides and 6 percent terpenes.

151. DON'T TAKE GINKGO IF . . .

Considered a brain-friendly herb, for reasons scientists don't understand, ginkgo may interfere with antidepressant MAO-inhibitor drugs such as phenelzine sulfate (Nardil) or tranylcypromine (Parnate). If you're on heart medication and want to take ginkgo, consult your doctor first. And be sure to stick to the recommended dosage of 120 to 240 milligrams a day.

152. TRY "KOLA" FOR YOUR BRAIN

Because the ancient herb gotu kola helps rebuild energy reserves, it has become known as "food for the brain." Supposed to increase mental and physical strength, combat stress, and improve reflexes, it is popular in the West as a nerve tonic. Recent studies have shown that it improves circulation by increasing the flow of blood throughout the body and strengthening veins and capillaries. It is typically taken as capsules or an extract; follow the label's directions. Pregnant woman should not use this herb, nor should anyone with an overactive thyroid condition.

153. TRY ST. JOHN'S WORT

According to Michael T. Murray, ND, author of *Natural Alternatives to Prozac,* about twenty-five supervised, double-blind studies involving a total of 1,592 patients who received positive effects from St. John's wort reported that it improved psychological problems like depression, anxiety, and sleep disorders without side effects. In his book *Herbs for Your Health,* herbalist Stephen Foster warns that St. John's wort should primarily be used as a safer, nonaddictive antidepressant aid until the true causes of the depression are uncovered and treated properly. **Caution:** No one ever should treat depression lightly, and neither St. John's wort nor other herbal treatments should be used to replace prescription drugs being taken by people who have been diagnosed with clinical depression. Do not combine it with antidepressants and always consult your physician first.

154. TRY AN ASPIRIN SUBSTITUTE

There are two herbs that make good substitutes for aspirin: vervain and white willow bark. In fact, aspirin was originally created from white willow bark and meadowsweet; meadowsweet's Latin name *Spirea* provided the *spirin* in *aspirin.* Chemically, vervain is different from aspirin while willow bark contains aspirin-like compounds. However, they do not upset the stomach. Both herbs are useful to relieve pain and inflammation. **Caution**: They should be taken in standard doses as advised by the manufacturer and should not be used by pregnant women.

155. TRY FEVERFEW FOR MIGRAINES

In 1985, *Lancet,* the prestigious British medical journal, published an article that reported that extracts of feverfew inhibited the release of two substances considered to bring on migraine attacks—serotonin from platelets and prostaglandin from white blood cells. However, it is important to note that feverfew does not actually *cure* migraine—it only helps prevent or lessen it. Long-term use has not been shown to be a problem, although more research is needed. It can take several months of regular use for feverfew to work. When using capsules or tablets, be sure to read the label carefully; some brands contain only trace amounts of the pure herb. Also, consult with your physician regarding dosage.

156. TRY HERBS TO RELIEVE YOUR STRESS

Here are some herbal remedies:

▶ Linden reduces nervous tension and helps prevent arteriosclerosis.
▶ Pasque flower contains nervine and anodyne with sedative action. It is useful for nervous and sexual problems.
▶ Skullcap acts as a relaxant and restorative for the central nervous system. It is good for nervous debility.
▶ Wood betony is a sedative that acts to calm the nervous system by soothing fearfulness and invigorating exhaustion.
▶ Vervain calms nerves and has a tonic effect on the liver.

157. TRY RAINFOREST HERBS

Rainforest plants are complex chemical storehouses that contain many undiscovered biodynamic compounds with unrealized potential for use in modern medicine. Following are some of the most important healing medicinal plants, as listed in *Herbal Secrets of the Rainforest* by Leslie Taylor. You can also learn more by reading *Kava: Medicine Hunting in Paradise* by Chris Kilham, who conducts research on medicinal plants around the world.

▶ Acerola—Contains vitamin C. Promotes a healthy circulatory system.
▶ Alcachofra (Artichoke)—Detoxifies the liver. Digestive stimulant. Eat whole vegetable or buy standard extract from health food store.
▶ Boldo—Detoxifies the liver; rids liver of fat. Promotes healthy bile flow.
▶ Cat's Claw—Aids intestinal immune system and chronic arthritis.
▶ Damiana—Used for hormone regulation in men and women.
▶ Guarana—Promotes health and energy.

- Muira Puama—Relieves stress; regulates hormones; promotes healthy central nervous system; general health tonic.
- Suma—Regulates female hormones; strengthens immune system; aids in regulation of cholesterol. Also used as general health tonic. Also known as Brazilian ginseng.

158. SUPPORT THE RAINFOREST

It is estimated that nearly half of the world's estimated ten million species of plants, animals, and microorganisms will be destroyed or severely threatened over the next quarter of a century due to rainforest deforestation. Harvard's Pulitzer prize–winning biologist Edward O. Wilson estimates that we are losing 137 plant, animal, and insect species every single day. That's 50,000 species a year! Rainforests currently provide sources for ¼ of today's medicines, and 70 percent of the plants found to have anticancer properties are found *only* in the rainforest. The rainforest and its immense undiscovered biodiversity hold the key to unlocking tomorrow's cures for devastating diseases. Get involved—it's good for your brain and your pain. Write to Rainforest Alliance, 665 Broadway, Suite 500, New York, NY 10012 or visit *www.rainforest-alliance.org* for more information on how you can help. Passion feeds your soul and your brain.

159. TRY NATURAL HERBS AND PLANTS TO COMBAT CHRONIC PROBLEMS

Many natural herbs and plants have been identified and used to improve certain conditions. Consider the following:

- Cholesterol Reduction—Angelica, black cohosh, hawthorn, hawthorn and walnut (combination), and mistletoe
- Energy—Fo-ti, ginseng, gotu kola

- Fatigue—capsicum (cayenne), ginseng, American ginseng and red deer antler (combination), gotu kola, and oats
- Headache—Chamomile, feverfew, hops, peppermint plus catnip (tea for headaches of stomach origin), red sage, skullcap, spearmint (tea), white willow, and wood betony
- Hypertension—cayenne (capsicum), garlic, glucomannan, hawthorn berries, hibiscus flowers, hops, lady's slipper, passionflower, skullcap, and valerian
- Insomnia—catnip, chamomile, hops, lady's slipper, skullcap, and valerian root
- Memory—astragalus, calamus, cayenne, dong quai, ginkgo biloba leaf extract, ginger, ginseng, gotu kola, and red deer antler
- Mental Health—cayenne, ginseng, and gotu kola
- Nervousness—betony, catnip, chamomile, european vervain, hops, lady's slipper, mistletoe, passionflower, pulsatilla, red sage (for nervous headache), skullcap, and valerian
- Stress—alfalfa, chamomile, ginseng, gotu kola, hops, kelp, lady's slipper, passionflower, and valerian

160. DRINK HAWTHORN TEA

Hawthorn berries have been scientifically proven to lower high blood pressure, a prime risk factor for heart disease. It's also an excellent antioxidant that eliminates free radicals, the dangerous agents that roam the body and can cause damage to blood vessels, leading to atherosclerosis. Hawthorn also contains rutin, a substance that reduces the formation of plaque, a buildup of which can block blood flow and possibly lead to stroke or a heart attack. Hawthorn is also effective against arrhythmia, a heart rhythm disturbance. This herb has been shown to promote overall improvement in heart health and blood flow, ease angina and shortness of breath, and reduce ankle swelling.

161. MAKE HERBAL TEA

Herbal teas have been brewed for thousands of years. They often boost your health in subtle and not-so-subtle ways. Here are a few varieties to consider:

- ▶ Bilberry tea—Aids circulation
- ▶ Catnip tea—Relaxant and mild depressant
- ▶ Chicory tea—Normalizes liver function
- ▶ Cinnamon tea—Clears the brain and improves thought processes
- ▶ Dandelion tea—Improves liver function and kidney function
- ▶ Ginseng tea—Natural tonic for a "lift"
- ▶ Hawthorn berries tea—Energizing to the elderly
- ▶ Jasmine tea—Mild nerve sedative
- ▶ Maté tea—Tones muscles, especially the smooth muscles of the heart
- ▶ Sage tea—Improves brain nourishment, known as the "thinker's tea"

Caution: If you are pregnant or have a medical condition such as high blood pressure, check with your doctor before drinking any herbal tea. ✳

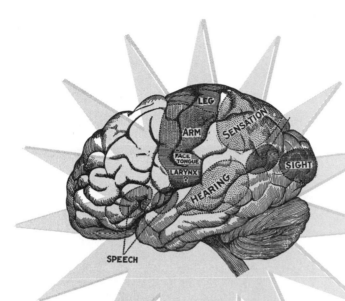

7

NOURISH
YOUR BRAIN
WITH MINERALS

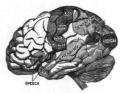

NOURISH YOUR BRAIN WITH MINERALS

Twenty-two minerals are essential to good health.

162. UNDERSTAND THE IMPORTANCE OF MINERALS

Minerals are different from vitamins in that they do not contain carbon, which makes them inorganic compounds. They cannot be destroyed as easily as vitamins by heat or poor handling. Minerals help to both regulate body processes and give your body structure. Just like vitamins, minerals are only needed in small amounts. More than sixty minerals are found in the body. Of those, twenty-two are considered essential to good health. Minerals are divided into two categories: major and trace. As the names imply, major minerals are required in larger amounts than trace.

163. UNDERSTAND HOW MINERALS WORK

All minerals are absorbed into your intestines and then are transported and stored in your body in various ways. Some minerals pass directly into your bloodstream, which transports them to the cells; the excess passes out of the body through the urine. Other minerals, such as calcium, attach to proteins and become part of your body structure (in the case of calcium, the bones). Because these types of minerals are stored, large amounts taken for a long period of time can be harmful.

164. TAKE POTASSIUM

Potassium is an electrolyte that works closely with its counterparts, chloride and sodium. Over 95 percent of potassium is in the body's cells and helps regulate the flow of fluids and minerals in and out of the body's cells. It also helps maintain normal blood pressure, maintain heart and kidney function, and transmit nerve impulses and contraction of muscles. Studies have also shown that potassium may also reduce the risk of high blood pressure and stroke. Potassium is very important in converting blood sugar into glycogen, the storage form of blood sugar in your muscles and liver. Potassium is widely available in foods, but chronic diarrhea, vomiting, diabetic acidosis, kidney disease, or prolonged use of laxatives or diuretics could cause a deficiency. Most people excrete excess potassium in their urine. If the excess cannot be excreted—for instance, in the case of someone with kidney disease—it can cause heart problems. Some experts recommend a higher intake, around 3,500 milligrams per day, to help protect against high blood pressure.

165. CHOOSE FOODS RICH IN POTASSIUM

A diet low in fat and cholesterol and rich in foods containing potassium, magnesium, and calcium—such as fruits, vegetables, legumes, and dairy foods—has shown evidence of reducing blood pressure. Potassium-rich foods include fresh meat, poultry, fish, figs, lentils, kidney beans, black beans, baked potatoes (with skin), avocados, orange juice, cantaloupes, bananas, and cooked spinach.

166. UNDERSTAND HOW SODIUM WORKS

Sodium is also an electrolyte that works closely with potassium and chloride. In contrast to potassium, most of the body's sodium is found outside the cells in blood and other body fluids. There is a pump in the membrane of all cells that flushes sodium out of and brings potassium into the cell. If sodium is not pumped out properly, water accumulates in the cell, causing it to swell. Sodium helps relax your muscles (including your heart muscle), transmit nerve impulses, and regulate blood pressure. Sodium can contribute to hypertension by raising blood pressure. A sodium deficiency is unlikely except in cases of prolonged diarrhea, vomiting, fasting, starvation, or kidney problems. Healthy people excrete excess sodium. The rest comes from table salt and small amounts that occur naturally in foods. There is no RDA or DRI for sodium; however, the amount considered safe and adequate is 500 milligrams daily.

167. REDUCE YOUR SODIUM

In the United States, the typical diet contains excessive amounts of sodium. Processed foods are one of the biggest contributors to our sodium intake. Healthy American adults should reduce their sodium intake to no more than 2,400 milligrams per day. This is almost 1¼ teaspoons of sodium chloride or table salt each day.

168. SEEK THE PROPER BALANCE

It is important to have a proper balance of both potassium and sodium in the diet. Studies have indicated a possible link between a diet high in sodium and low in potassium with an increased risk of cancer, heart disease, high blood pressure, and stroke. On the other hand, a diet high in potassium and low in sodium may help to protect or decrease the risk for these health problems.

169. UNDERSTAND HOW CHLORIDE WORKS

Chloride is another electrolyte that works closely with potassium and sodium. Chloride also helps regulate body fluids in and out of body cells. Chloride joins sodium in surrounding the fluids outside the cells. This mineral is a component of stomach acid that helps with the digestion of food and the absorption of nutrients. Chloride also helps to transmit nerve impulses. As stated earlier, many salt substitutes also contain chloride in the form of potassium chloride. Deficiencies are rare.

170. TAKE MAGNESIUM

This mineral is an absolute must for proper brain function in that it aids neuron metabolism, helps reduce brain damage from ischemia (a lack of blood flow to the brain), and boosts the effectiveness of certain antioxidants. Magnesium may also play a role in the prevention of Alzheimer's disease, since studies show that the brains of most AD patients are magnesium-deficient, but excessively high in calcium. (In healthy brains, the two minerals have a relatively equal ratio.) Every cell in the body needs magnesium. Magnesium is a requirement for more than 300 body enzymes, body chemicals that regulate all kinds of body functions. This mineral helps maintain normal nerve and muscle function, keeps heart rhythm steady, and helps keep bones strong. Deficiency can result from an increase in urine output—like that caused by diuretics—poorly controlled diabetes, and alcoholism. Too much magnesium is not harmful unless the mineral is not excreted properly due to disorders such as kidney disease. The UL for magnesium is 350 mg per day for adults over eighteen.

171. CHOOSE FOODS RICH IN MAGNESIUM

Magnesium can be found in a wide variety of foods. The best sources include legumes, almonds, avocados, toasted wheat germ, wheat bran, fish, seafood, fruits, fruit juice, pumpkin seeds, and whole grains. Green vegetables, especially cooked spinach, can be good sources too.

172. ADD MAGNESIUM TO LOWER BLOOD PRESSURE

Higher blood levels of magnesium have been associated with lower risk of coronary heart disease, and higher magnesium intakes have been linked to a lower risk of stroke. Studies show that magnesium may also play an important role in regulating blood pressure. The recent DASH study (Dietary Approaches to Stop Hypertension) suggested that a diet high in calcium, magnesium, and potassium, and lower in sodium and fat, could lower high blood pressure significantly. The Joint National Committee on Prevention, Detection, Evaluation and Treatment of High Blood Pressure recommends maintaining an adequate magnesium intake to prevent and manage high blood pressure. Try increasing your consumption to 410 to 420 milligrams per day.

173. ADD MAGNESIUM TO COMBAT MIGRAINES

People who suffer from migraine headaches may also be magnesium-deficient. In one study, migraine patients who took 600 milligrams of magnesium per day for 12 weeks went from three attacks per month down to two. Migraine patients who were given the placebo noticed no change in the number of headaches.

174. DON'T DEPLETE YOUR PHOSPHORUS

Phosphorus is second only to calcium in terms of its abundance in the body. Phosphorus contributes to the structure of bones and teeth. It helps generate energy in every cell in the body and acts as the main regulator in converting dietary carbohydrates, protein, and fat to energy. Phosphorus is vital to growth, maintenance, and repair of all body tissue. This mineral also helps activate B vitamins and is a component of the storage form of energy in the body. A deficiency of phosphorus is very rare, but absorption can be reduced by the long-term and excessive use of antacids containing aluminum hydroxide.

175. CHOOSE FOODS RICH IN PHOSPHORUS

Phosphorus is found in almost all food groups. The best sources are protein-rich foods like milk, meat, poultry, fish, and eggs. Legumes and nuts are also good sources. Whole grains can also be good sources of phosphorus.

176. TAKE CALCIUM

Calcium's primary function is to help build and maintain bones and teeth. In addition, calcium helps blood clot, helps your muscles contract and your heart beat, helps regulate blood pressure, plays a role in normal nerve function and nerve transmission, and helps regulate the secretion of hormones and digestive enzymes. Calcium works in conjunction with vitamin D, phosphorus, and fluoride to help promote strong and healthy bones. Vitamin D is necessary for the absorption of calcium in the body. Low levels of calcium intake can lead to osteomalacia (softening of the bones) and an increased risk of osteoporosis. Calcium has a UL set at 2,500 mg per day for adults and children. When consuming supplements up to this amount, no adverse effects are likely. However, higher doses over an extended period of time may cause kidney stones and poor kidney function as well as reduce the absorption of other minerals such as iron and zinc.

177. CHOOSE FOODS RICH IN CALCIUM

Some of the best sources of calcium are foods in the dairy group, such as milk, cheese, and yogurt. In addition, some dark green leafy vegetables, such as broccoli, spinach, kale, and collards, are good sources. Other good sources include fish with edible bones, such as sardines and salmon, as well as calcium-fortified soymilk, tofu made with calcium, shelled almonds, cooked dried beans, calcium-fortified cereals, and calcium-fortified orange juice.

178. ADD CALCIUM TO COMBAT HIGH BLOOD PRESSURE

In a review of 22 studies, calcium supplementation was found to moderately reduce blood pressure in adults with hypertension, or high blood pressure, but had little effect on people with normal blood pressure. Calcium is found in dairy products and dark leafy vegetables, such as kale, collards, turnip greens, and broccoli. Take a minimum of 1,000 and a maximum of 2,000 milligrams a day. Experts recommend a two-to-one ratio of calcium to magnesium. If you regularly supplement with extra calcium, be sure to increase your magnesium intake, too.

179. UNDERSTAND TRACE MINERALS

Minerals that are needed in smaller amounts than the major minerals are referred to as trace minerals or trace elements. Even though our bodies only require a small amount of these minerals, they are still very important to proper health. Most trace minerals are needed in amounts of less than 20 mg per day. There are no RDAs, DRIs, or safe and adequate ranges set for these minerals because not enough is known about what the body requires for proper health and functioning. A healthy, varied, and balanced diet is the best way to ensure you consume safe and adequate amounts of these other trace minerals.

180. PROTECT YOUR CELLS WITH SELENIUM

This very powerful antioxidant benefits the brain by preventing oxidation of fat. Why is this important? It's important because more than half of the brain is composed of a type of fat. By inhibiting oxidation, selenium slows age-related brain deterioration and preserves cognitive function. Selenium also benefits the immune system, and some studies suggest that it improves circulation throughout the body. Because selenium levels tend to decline with age, older people should take selenium supplements in addition to adding selenium-rich foods to their diets.

Selenium also works with glutathione peroxidase to keep potentially damaging free radicals under control. In Japan, where people traditionally consume about 500 micrograms of selenium a day, the cancer rate is nearly five times lower than in countries where daily selenium intake is less. There is no established RDA for selenium, though men and women can safely consume between 50 and 200 micrograms daily, not exceeding 400 mcg per day for adults over eighteen.

181. EAT FOODS RICH IN SELENIUM
Natural sources of selenium include broccoli, cabbage, celery, cucumbers, garlic, onions, kidney, liver, chicken, whole-grain foods, seafood, and milk.

182. DON'T OVERDO SELENIUM
Selenium can become toxic if 700 micrograms are consumed on a daily basis.

183. PROTECT YOUR DNA WITH ZINC
This mineral aids the brain as part of a metabolic process that eliminates harmful free radicals. It also strengthens neuronal membranes for greater protection and helps get rid of lead, which can enter the brain through automobile exhaust and other sources and adversely affect mental function. Zinc is part of the molecular structure of dozens of important enzymes, is a component of the insulin that regulates our energy supply, and works with red blood cells to transport waste carbon dioxide from body tissue to the lungs, where it is expelled. Zinc is also vital to the production of the RNA and DNA that oversee the division, growth, and repair of

the body's cells; helps preserve our sense of taste and smell; and aids in wound healing. Dietary sources of zinc include beef, herring, seafood, pork, poultry, milk, soybeans, and whole grains. The RDA for zinc is 15 milligrams, not to exceed 40 mg per day for adults over eighteen years of age. Women who are pregnant may want to take an additional 5 milligrams of zinc daily, and women who are breast-feeding an extra 10 milligrams daily.

184. EAT COPPER-RICH FOODS

Copper is found in all the tissues in the body but is concentrated in the brain, heart, kidney, and liver. It helps the body make hemoglobin (needed to carry oxygen to red blood cells) and red blood cells by aiding in the absorption of iron in the body. Copper is part of many enzymes in the body and helps produce energy in cells. In addition, copper helps make hormones that regulate a variety of body functions, including heartbeat, blood pressure, and wound healing. Most deficiencies are due to a genetic problem or from too much zinc. Copper is found mostly in organ meats, especially liver, and in seafood, nuts, and seeds. It can also be found in poultry, legumes, and dark green leafy vegetables.

185. INCREASE YOUR INTAKE OF CHROMIUM

Chromium is a mineral that helps the body metabolize fat, convert blood sugar into energy, and make insulin work more efficiently. In addition to the benefits already noted, several recent studies have also shown that chromium protects the heart by lowering serum cholesterol levels and triglycerides. Chromium is derived primarily from our diet. Rich sources include whole-grain foods, eggs, broccoli, orange juice, grape juice, seafood, dairy products, and many different types of meat. Trivalent chromium, the form in most chromium supplements, is extremely safe.

186. EAT FOODS RICH IN IRON

Almost two-thirds of the iron in your body is found in hemoglobin, the protein in red blood cells that carries oxygen to your body's tissues. Smaller amounts are found in myoglobin, a protein that helps supply oxygen to muscle. About 15 percent of your body's iron is stored for future needs and activated when dietary intake is inadequate. Iron is also needed for a strong immune system and for energy production. In the United States, iron deficiency is one of the most common nutrient deficiencies. Iron deficiency can lead to anemia, fatigue, and infections. Foods rich in iron include beef liver, fortified cereals, lean red meats, nuts, seeds, poultry, bran, spinach, salmon, legumes, lentils, whole-wheat bread, and wheat germ. It is best to seek the advice of your doctor before taking an iron supplement.

187. KNOW WHEN YOU MAY NEED MORE IRON

Certain types of people are at higher risk for iron deficiency and should be screened periodically:

► Infants and children, because of their growth and choosy eating habits
► Adolescents, especially girls who have started their menstrual cycle, who consume a junk food diet
► Women who are pregnant, because they are supporting their needs as well as the baby's
► The elderly population because of poor dietary intake and decreased iron absorption due to aging
► Women of childbearing age who experience excessive menstrual bleeding because they lose iron-rich blood each month
► Strict vegetarians who eat only plant foods, because the iron in these foods is not absorbed as well as the iron in animal products (Consuming vitamin

C–rich foods at meals can help enhance your body's ability to absorb plant-based iron.)

- ► People who abuse crash diets and people suffering from eating disorders
- ► A person who loses an excessive amount of blood through surgery or other incident

188. BE AWARE OF DANGERS ASSOCIATED WITH IRON

Your body usually maintains normal iron status by controlling the amount of iron absorbed from food, but iron can build up and become harmful in people who have a genetic disorder called hemochromatosis. This disorder, which usually occurs in men, causes excessive iron to accumulate in soft tissue. The result can be heart problems and other abnormalities. **Caution**: In children, large amounts of iron can have serious consequences. Keep iron supplements and other adult nutrient supplements out of the reach of children. Children should get immediate medical attention if they take an overdose of iron supplements.

189. DON'T OVERDO IRON

Iron supplementation may be indicated when an iron deficiency is diagnosed and when diet alone cannot restore bodily iron content to normal levels within an acceptable time frame. Taking iron supplements can cause side effects such as nausea, vomiting, constipation, diarrhea, dark-colored stools, and abdominal distress. To minimize these side effects, take only what your doctor recommends and take the supplement in divided doses and with food.

190. MEET YOUR DAILY BETA

Beta carotene is a fat-soluble antioxidant that your body converts to vitamin A (retinol) and is present in liver, egg yolk, milk, butter, spinach, carrots, squash, broccoli, yams, tomatoes, cantaloupe, peaches, and grains. Because beta caro-tene is converted to vitamin A by the body, there is no set requirement, but making sure you eat beta-rich foods boosts your health.

191. INDULGE IN TRYPTOPHAN (5-HTP)

The body makes a chemical known as 5-HTP from the tryptophan we get from food. The 5-HTP used in supplements comes from the seeds of an African plant *(Griffonia simplicifolia)*. In our bodies, 5-HTP quickly becomes serotonin, a neurotransmitter (a chemical that carries messages to and from the brain) that affects sleep cycles, appetite, and mood. Extra tryptophan in our diets leads to extra serotonin in our brains, which is why the supplements are touted as a sleep aid and mood-lifter, among other things. Foods that provide tryptophan (5-HTP) include roasted white turkey, ground beef, cottage cheese, chicken thighs, eggnog, milk, and almonds.

192. ADD COENZYME Q_{10}

CoQ_{10} has been shown to be useful in alleviating the effects of abnormalities involv-ing the heart's ability to contract and pump blood effectively, such as congestive heart failure and a number of heart muscle diseases. Coenzyme Q_{10} also appears to protect vitamin E, which helps prevent the oxidation of low-density lipoprotein (LDL, or "bad" cholesterol). It's believed that oxidized LDL can lead to plaque buildup, clogged arteries, and an increased risk of heart attack or stroke. CoQ_{10} may reduce the ability of blood to clot, thereby decreasing the chance of a blood clot getting stuck in a clogged artery and causing a heart attack or stroke. Other heart-related conditions for which CoQ_{10} supplementation shows promise include hypertension and heart valve replacement. To bulk up on CoQ_{10} eat sardines, mackerel, nuts, organ meats, beef, broccoli, chicken, oranges, salmon, or trout.

193. TAKE FISH OIL CAPSULES

Several studies have looked at the role of omega-3 fatty acids in blood pressure. The findings indicate that high doses of fish oil can reduce both systolic (the top number in a blood pressure reading) and diastolic (the bottom number) blood pressure in individuals with mildly elevated blood pressure. Some experts believe it may be the DHA component of fish oil that is exerting the protective effects.

194. ASK YOUR DOCTOR ABOUT SAMe

SAMe (pronounced "Sammy") is a form of the amino acid methionine that occurs naturally in the body and is used for many essential functions, including making cartilage. SAMe appears to increase the levels of certain neurotransmitters, and may thereby affect moods and emotions. In nine studies, SAMe compared favorably with antidepressant drugs, including imipramine, amitryptaline, and clomipramine. Some researchers have found that SAMe supplementation has improved mood disorders, without the side effects of other antidepressants (such as weight gain, headaches, sleep disturbances, and sexual dysfunction). And, SAMe works faster than some prescription antidepressants, often in four to ten days compared with two to six weeks for drugs.

195. DON'T TAKE SAMe IF . . .

When it comes to taking SAMe as a relief from psychological problems, never attempt to self-medicate—always consult your doctor. Absolutely do not take SAMe when you are already taking drugs for bipolar depression, obsessive compulsive disorder, or addictive tendencies, as it has been known to worsen symptoms.

196. BOLSTER YOUR AMINO ACIDS

Amino acids, simply put, are organic compounds that help make proteins and are essential to human metabolism. Though they don't receive nearly as much mention in nutrition discussions as vitamins and minerals, they are just as necessary to our health—particularly for brain function. Let's take a closer look at some of the most important amino acids in terms of maintaining mental acuity:

▶ ***Arginine.*** This amino acid is partially converted into a chemical known as spermine, which is believed to help the brain process memory. Low levels of spermine often signal age-related memory loss.

▶ ***Choline.*** The brain uses this amino acid to manufacture a memory-related neurotransmitter called acetylcholine. Older people are encouraged to take choline supplements because as we age we tend to produce less acetylcholine, putting us at greater risk of memory impairment. Dietary sources of choline include cabbage, cauliflower, eggs, peanuts, and lecithin.

▶ ***Glutamine.*** This amino acid is a precursor of a calming neurotransmitter known as GABA. It also helps improve clarity of thought and boosts alertness by assisting in the manufacture of glutamic acid, a compound known for its ability to eliminate metabolic wastes in the brain.

▶ ***Methionine.*** Like glutamine, this amino acid helps cleanse the brain of damaging metabolic wastes. It is an effective antioxidant and helps reduce brain levels of dangerous heavy metals such as mercury. ✳

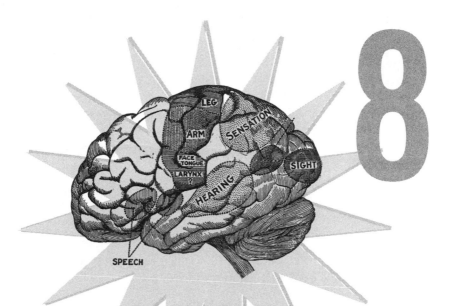

8

REPLENISH YOUR BRAIN WITH VITAMINS

111

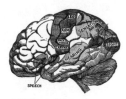

REPLENISH YOUR BRAIN WITH VITAMINS

It's best to get vitamins you need from your diet.

197. UNDERSTAND MICRONUTRIENTS

A healthy diet consists not only of optimal portions of macronutrients (food) but also recommended levels of essential micronutrients. Micronutrients include vitamins and minerals. Vitamins are labeled as "micro" nutrients because they are only needed in small amounts to do their jobs properly. Don't let the "micro" fool you, though, good things come in small packages! The micronutrients are just as essential as the macronutrients in helping to keep your body functioning properly.

198. UNDERSTAND HOW VITAMINS WORK

Vitamins are natural substances that are necessary for almost every process in the body. Micronutrients help trigger thousands of chemical reactions essential to maintaining good health. Most of these reactions are linked because one triggers another. A missing vitamin or a deficiency of a certain vitamin anywhere in the linked chain can cause a collapse, with health problems being the result. Vitamins are organic compounds (or compounds that contain carbon) that are required in small amounts and are necessary to promote growth, health, and life.

112

199. UNDERSTAND WHY YOU NEED VITAMINS

Vitamins are produced by living material such as plants and animals. Most vitamins are not made by the body in sufficient amounts to maintain health, so must be obtained through a person's diet. Vitamins are classified into two groups: fat-soluble and water-soluble. Unlike macronutrients, vitamins do not provide calories or directly supply energy, but they do assist the calories in carbohydrates, proteins, and fats to produce energy. Consuming macronutrients (carbohydrates, proteins, and fat) supplies the thirteen vitamins that the body requires. Vitamins are found in a wide variety of foods, with some foods being better sources than others. For this reason, eating a wide variety of foods ensures a better intake of vitamins.

200. CONSIDER DIETARY SUPPLEMENTS

Eating a healthy and varied diet can provide the ideal mixture of vitamins, minerals, and other nutrients. However, even people with the best intentions sometimes fall short of their nutritional needs. Today the definition of dietary supplements covers vitamins, minerals, fiber, herbs and other botanicals, amino acids, concentrates, and extracts. The body more readily absorbs nutrients when they come from the foods we eat so, ideally, it is best to get all of your necessary nutrients from your diet. Nevertheless, some people do need assistance to receive their required daily allowances.

201. EVALUATE YOUR DIET

There are some people who may benefit from taking supplements. Look at your diet and ask yourself whether you do these things on most days:

▶ Eat 6 to 11 servings of grains (bread, cereal, rice, pasta, and other grain foods).
▶ Eat at least 3 servings of vegetables.

- Eat at least 2 servings of fruit.
- Eat 2 or more servings of low-fat or fat-free dairy products, such as milk, yogurt, or cheese.
- Eat 2 to 3 servings of lean meat, poultry, fish, dried beans, eggs, or nuts.
- Eat a varied diet.
- Eat at least three well-balanced meals.

If you fall short on any of these behaviors, you may benefit from taking a daily multivitamin and mineral supplement. Supplements are not meant to take the place of any food group or meal, but they can help supplement what you may not get every single day. Your top goal should be to include all of these options as often as possible. If you don't, choose one food group at a time and try to gradually improve your daily eating pattern. Aim to at least eat the minimum number of servings each day.

202. MAKE SURE YOUR NEEDS ARE BEING MET

Other people who may want to consider a multivitamin and mineral supplement include the following:

- Strict vegetarians may need extra calcium, iron, zinc, vitamin B_{12}, and vitamin D.
- Women with heavy menstrual bleeding may need to replace iron each month.
- Women who are pregnant or breastfeeding need more of some nutrients. Be sure to speak with your doctor first.
- Menopausal women can benefit from calcium supplements.
- People on a low-calorie diet can benefit from supplements.
- People over sixty years of age may benefit because they may have a decreased absorption of numerous vitamins and minerals.

- ► People who suffer from lactose intolerance or milk allergies may be advised to take a vitamin D and a calcium supplement.
- ► People with impaired nutrient absorption may be instructed by their doctor to take a supplement.
- ► People who regularly smoke and/or drink alcohol should consider a supplement because these habits interfere with the body's ability to absorb and use certain vitamins and minerals.

203. CONSULT YOUR DOCTOR ABOUT VITAMINS

While you are relatively safe taking a multivitamin, when you want to boost your intake of specific vitamins, it is always wise to run it past your doctor. If you take medication, it is particularly important to make sure elevated levels of vitamins will not adversely affect the medication. Some vitamins can be toxic when taken in huge doses.

204. CHOOSE WISELY

If you are going to take a supplement, it is important to take the time to choose the product that is right for you. Follow some of these tips to help you choose a dietary supplement:

- ► Pick a supplement that contains at least twenty vitamins and minerals essential for good health and no more than 150 percent of the Reference Daily Intakes (RDI) for each nutrient.
- ► Choose a supplement tailored to your needs, whether it is age, gender, or medical status.

- Don't be lured by extra ingredients such as choline, inositol, herbs, enzymes, or PABA. These add no proven nutritional benefits and only make the supplements more expensive.
- Check the expiration date on the bottle. Vitamins are especially perishable. After the expiration date, they are probably not very potent.
- Take the supplement only as directed on the bottle or prescribed by your doctor.
- Keep all supplements out of the reach of children.

205. FAMILIARIZE YOURSELF WITH LABELING PRACTICES

Before learning why each vitamin is important and how much you need, it is crucial to understand how these values are generated. In the United States, the Food and Nutrition Board of the National Academy of Sciences/National Research Council is responsible for establishing and updating nutrition guidelines. The Recommended Daily Allowances, or RDAs, have always been the benchmark for adequate nutritional intake in the United States. The RDAs are based on scientific evidence. They reflect the amount of a nutrient that is sufficient to meet the requirement of 97 to 98 percent of healthy individuals in a particular life stage and gender group.

206. FAMILIARIZE YOURSELF WITH CHANGES IN LABELING

Because scientific knowledge of the relationship between nutrition and health has broadened so much, the Food and Nutrition Board partnered with Health Canada in the late 1990s. Together, the agencies developed a new approach called Dietary Reference Intakes (DRIs). DRIs represent an approach that serves to optimize health instead of just preventing nutritional deficiencies as the RDAs have. DRIs incorporate an average of three types of reference values:

- ► Estimated Average Requirement (EAR)
- ► Recommended Daily Allowance (RDA) or Adequate Intake (AI)
- ► Tolerable Upper Intake Level (UL)

The EAR is a daily nutrient intake value that is estimated to meet the requirements of half of the healthy individuals in a life stage and gender group. The RDA is the dietary intake level that is sufficient to meet the nutrient requirements of nearly all (97 to 98 percent) individuals in a specified group. The AIs are a recommended intake value based on observed or experimentally determined estimates of nutrient intake by a group of healthy people that are assumed to be adequate. They are basically used when there is not enough information available to establish an RDA. The Tolerable Upper Intake Level (UL) is the highest daily recommended intake of a nutrient that is unlikely to pose risks of adverse health effects to almost all of the individuals in a specified group.

207. KNOW WHAT YOUR BRAIN NEEDS

Your brain needs just as many vitamins as the rest of your body does, and it gets them from the bloodstream. When vitamin absorption is reduced or impeded as a result of a poor diet or an illness, the brain is one of the first organs to feel it. We'll go through a quick rundown of some of the more essential vitamins needed for long-term brain health.

- ► *Vitamin A.* This antioxidant helps protect brain cells from harmful free radicals and benefits the circulatory system so blood flow to the brain remains strong.
- ► *Vitamin B$_{12}$.* An estimated 25 percent of people between ages sixty and seventy are deficient in this essential nutrient, as are nearly 40 percent of people

eighty and older. A B₁₂ deficiency may be mistaken for an age-related decline in mental function, including memory loss and a reduction in reasoning skills. To hedge your bet, take a multivitamin tablet daily.

- ▶ *Vitamin B₆.* This important vitamin helps convert sugar into glucose, which the brain needs for fuel. It also benefits general circulation, which can improve memory. Older people need substantially more B_6 than younger people, so make sure your diet is packed with this nutrient.

- ▶ *Vitamin B₁.* Like B_{12}, this nutrient is a potent antioxidant. It is also required for numerous metabolic processes within the brain and peripheral nervous system.

- ▶ *Folic Acid.* This nutrient, also a member of the B vitamin family, is known to aid cerebral circulation by inhibiting narrowing of the arteries in the neck. Studies also suggest that daily supplements of folic acid can reduce the likelihood of certain age-related psychiatric problems, including dementia.

- ▶ *Vitamin C.* This well-known antioxidant is extremely important for proper brain function and, as such, is found in much higher levels within the brain than other parts of the body. In addition to boosting the effectiveness of other antioxidants, vitamin C is an essential ingredient in the manufacture of several neurotransmitters such as dopamine and acetylcholine. In short, a daily dose of vitamin C can boost and maintain mental acuity. So important is vitamin C to proper brain function that it is being evaluated as a possible nutritional preventative for Alzheimer's disease.

- ▶ *Vitamin E.* Yet another important antioxidant, vitamin E also restores damaged neurotransmitter receptor sites on neurons. This means that vitamin E both prevents age-related brain deterioration and also reverses a specific aspect of that breakdown. There is also evidence that vitamin E can prevent the onset of Alzheimer's disease and slow its progression once it develops, and that a combination of vitamin E and the mineral selenium can dramatically improve mood and cognitive function in older patients. In addition, vitamin E can help reduce risk of heart disease, stroke, and certain types of cancer.

208. KNOW WHY EXCESSIVE FAT-SOLUBLE VITAMINS CAN BE DANGEROUS

Out of the thirteen vitamins your body needs, four of them are fat-soluble vitamins. These four vitamins are vitamin A, D, E, and K. Fat-soluble vitamins dissolve in fat and are carried throughout your body attached to body chemicals made with fat. This is one important reason you need moderate amounts of fat in your daily diet. The body can store fat-soluble vitamins in its fat stores and in the liver. For this reason, consuming too much of a fat-soluble vitamin, usually in a supplemental form, for a long period of time can be harmful.

209. TAKE VITAMIN A

Vitamin A promotes healthy vision (especially night vision), growth and health of cells and tissues, bone growth, and tooth development. Vitamin A also helps protect you from infection by keeping mucous membranes in your mouth, stomach, intestines, respiratory, and urinary tracts healthy and acts as a powerful antioxidant in the form of beta carotene.

There are several forms of vitamin A. Retinol is a form that is found in animal foods. It is readily available to the body and is known as preformed vitamin A. Another form of vitamin A is a group called carotenoids, which includes beta carotene. Beta carotene is the carotenoid most readily converted by the body to vitamin A. A significant deficiency of vitamin A can cause night blindness and other eye problems, dry and scaly skin, reproductive problems, and poor growth. Too much vitamin A (retinol) can lead to headaches, dry and scaly skin, bone and joint pain, liver damage, vomiting, loss of appetite, abnormal bone growth, nerve damage, and birth defects.

210. DON'T OVERDO VITAMIN A

When taking a supplement, make sure you are not taking more vitamin A (retinol) than you need for your age range and gender. You will find a breakdown of vitamin A into beta carotene and retinol on most supplement labels. Even though beta carotene is not toxic to the body, it is not recommended to take megadoses through supplements. Vitamin A has a UL set at 3,000 micrograms (mcg) or 10,000 IU (international units) per day for adults over eighteen. This is the highest daily recommended intake of vitamin A that is unlikely to pose risks of adverse health effects.

211. CHOOSE FOODS RICH IN VITAMIN A

Foods rich in vitamin A (retinol) include beef liver, eggs, milk fortified with vitamin A, other vitamin A–fortified foods, fish oil, margarine, and cheese. Foods rich in vitamin A (beta carotene) include sweet potatoes, carrots, kale, spinach, apricots, cantaloupe, broccoli, and winter squash.

212. TAKE VITAMIN D

Vitamin D promotes the absorption and use of two minerals: calcium and phosphorus. It helps deposit these two minerals in bones and teeth, making them stronger and healthier. The body can get vitamin D from two sources—food and the sun. This vitamin is known as the "sunshine vitamin" because the body can make vitamin D after sunlight hits the skin. The body's ability to produce vitamin D from sunlight diminishes with age; therefore, requirements increase for older adults. Not getting enough vitamin D throughout life can cause osteoporosis (or brittle bone disease) later in life.

213. DON'T OVERDO VITAMIN D

Because vitamin D is a fat-soluble vitamin, it can be toxic in larger doses. Toxicity can lead to kidney stones or damage, weakened muscles and bones, excessive bleeding, and other health problems. Levels high enough to cause health complications usually come from supplements, not from food or too much sunlight. If you take a supplement that includes vitamin D, make sure it does not contain more than you need for your age range and gender. Vitamin D has a UL set at 50 mcg or 2,000 IU per day for children and adults. There is no UL established for infants.

214. CHOOSE FOODS RICH IN VITAMIN D

Foods rich in vitamin D include fortified milk, cheese, egg yolks, salmon, margarine, mackerel, canned sardines, and fortified breakfast cereals.

215. TAKE VITAMIN E

Vitamin E is a natural substance found in many foods that acts as a natural antioxidant that diminishes free radicals. There is evidence to suggest that free radical damage to the neurons (nerve cells) is at least partially responsible for the development of Alzheimer's disease. Vitamin E has been shown to prevent free radical damage and delay memory deficits in animal studies. In a two-year study of people with Alzheimer's disease, progression of the disease was slowed when either 2,000 IU of vitamin E (alpha-tocopherol), a drug (10 milligrams Selegiline), or a combination of the two was taken daily. That said, large doses of vitamin E, when taken by healthy people, have not been shown to *prevent* Alzheimer's disease. As an antioxidant, vitamin E may affect aging, infertility, heart disease, and cancer. The mineral selenium enhances the antioxidant capabilities of vitamin E. Vitamin E is considered nontoxic, even over RDA levels. Vitamin E has a UL set at 1,000 mg per day for adults over eighteen.

216. CHOOSE FOODS RICH IN VITAMIN E

Foods rich in vitamin E include dried almonds, vegetable oils, salad dressing, nuts and seeds, wheat germ oil, peanut butter, and green leafy vegetables.

217. TAKE VITAMIN K

Vitamin K's primary function is to help make a protein, known as prothrombin, which is necessary for helping blood to clot. It also aids the body in making some other body proteins for blood, bones, and kidneys. Vitamin K is unique in that as well as being obtained from the diet, it is also made in the body from bacteria in the intestines. The prolonged use of antibiotics may affect your level of K because they destroy some bacteria in your intestines. There have been no reported problems in ingesting excess amounts of vitamin K, though moderation is still the best policy. Vitamin K has no established UL.

218. CHOOSE FOODS RICH IN VITAMIN K

Foods rich in vitamin K include turnip greens, green leafy vegetables like spinach or kale, broccoli, cabbage, beef liver, egg yolk, and wheat bran or wheat germ.

219. KNOW WHY WATER-SOLUBLE VITAMINS NEED REPLENISHMENT

Unlike the fat-soluble vitamins, water-soluble vitamins dissolve in water. These vitamins are carried in the bloodstream and for the most part are not stored in the body. In general, your body uses what it needs and excretes the rest through urine. For this reason it is important to regularly replenish these vitamins by eating a healthy and varied diet each day. Because water-soluble vitamins dissolve in water, they are much more easily destroyed in cooking and storing than the fat-soluble vitamins.

220. KNOW WHICH VITAMINS ARE WATER-SOLUBLE

The water-soluble vitamins consist of the B-complex vitamins and vitamin C. The B vitamins work together in converting carbohydrates, protein, and fats to energy, and many are found in the same foods. For this reason, poor intake of one B vitamin is usually associated with poor intake of other B vitamins.

221. TAKE VITAMIN B_1 (THIAMINE)

Thiamine is needed to help produce energy from the carbohydrates that you eat. It also is required for normal functioning of all body cells, especially nerves. A deficiency of thiamine can lead to beriberi, fatigue, mental confusion, loss of energy, nerve damage, muscle weakness, and impaired growth. Thiamine deficiency is very rare in the United States because most people consume plenty of grain products. Since thiamine is a water-soluble vitamin, the body excretes excess amounts that you consume. There are no known benefits to taking megadoses of thiamine, including the popular belief that it will help boost energy. Thiamine has no established UL.

222. CHOOSE FOODS RICH IN VITAMIN B_1

Foods rich in thiamine (vitamin B_1) include whole-grain foods, enriched-grain foods, fortified cereals, beef liver, pork, and wheat germ.

223. TAKE VITAMIN B_2 (RIBOFLAVIN)

Just like thiamine, riboflavin plays a key role in releasing energy from the macronutrients to all cells of the body. Riboflavin also helps change the amino acid (building blocks of protein) tryptophan into niacin, another B vitamin. Riboflavin is important in normal growth, production of certain hormones, formation of red blood cells, and in vision and skin health. A deficiency of riboflavin is unlikely but can cause eye disorders, dry and flaky skin, and burning and dryness of the mouth and tongue. The RDA for vitamin B_2 is 1.6 milligrams for men aged twenty-three to fifty, 1.4 milligrams for men fifty-one and older, 1.3 milligrams for women up to age twenty-two, and 1.2 milligrams for women twenty-three and older. Pregnant women require an additional 0.3 milligrams daily, and women who are breast-feeding require an extra 0.5 milligrams. There are no reported problems from consuming too much, but again, moderation is the best policy. Riboflavin has no established UL.

224. CHOOSE FOODS RICH IN VITAMIN B_2
Foods rich in riboflavin (vitamin B_2) include beef liver, milk, low-fat yogurt, cheese, enriched-grain foods, whole-grain foods, eggs, and green leafy vegetables.

225. TAKE VITAMIN B_3 (NIACIN)
More commonly known as niacin, vitamin B_3 is instrumental in maintaining the health of the skin, nerves, and digestive system. It also helps release energy from the food we eat, aids in the synthesis of DNA, and helps lower blood levels of cholesterol and triglycerides. The RDA for vitamin B_3 is 18 milligrams for men age twenty-three to fifty, 16 milligrams for men fifty and older, 14 milligrams for women fifteen to twenty-two, and 13 milligrams for women twenty-three and older. Women require an extra 2 milligrams of vitamin B_3 during pregnancy and an additional 4 milligrams while breastfeeding.

226. CHOOSE FOODS RICH IN VITAMIN B_3
Dietary sources of vitamin B_3 include whole grain foods, fortified cereal, lean meats, fish, poultry, peanuts, brewer's yeast, yogurt, and sunflower seeds.

227. DON'T OVERDO VITAMIN B₃

In large doses, niacin has been used as a cholesterol-lowering supplement. Because large doses can cause symptoms such as flushed skin, rashes, and even liver damage, this should only be done under a doctor's supervision. Niacin has a UL set at 35 mg per day for adults over eighteen.

228. TAKE VITAMIN B₆ (PYRIDOXINE)

Also known as pyridoxine and pyridoxal, vitamin B₆ plays a very important role in maintaining the body's immune system. It also helps the brain work properly, enables the body to resist stress, helps maintain the proper chemical balance in the body's fluids, works with other vitamins and minerals to supply the energy used by muscles, and is influential in cell growth. Vitamin B₆, in conjunction with folate (another B vitamin) and vitamin B₁₂, helps to lower blood levels of homocysteine, a risk factor for heart disease. The RDA for vitamin B₆ is 2.2 milligrams for men and 2.0 milligrams for women. Pregnant women need an additional 0.6 milligrams each day, and breastfeeding women need an extra 0.5 milligrams daily.

229. CHOOSE FOODS RICH IN VITAMIN B₆

Foods rich in B₆ include liver, beef, chicken, fish, bananas, carrots, lentils, rice, soybeans, whole grains, and avocados. Don't exceed 100 milligrams a day without checking with your doctor; excess can be toxic.

230. TAKE VITAMIN B₁₂ (COBALAMIN)

Vitamin B₁₂, in conjunction with folate (another B vitamin) and vitamin B₆, helps to lower blood levels of the amino acid homocysteine, a risk factor for heart disease. A lack of B₁₂ may cause a buildup of, or alter chemicals in the brain involved with mood. Other potential benefits of B_{12} supplements include the treatment of Alzheimer's disease and dementia, sleep disorders, and diabetic neuropathy. It is important to know that a deficiency of this vitamin can be hidden, and even progress, if extra folic acid is taken to treat or prevent anemia. There are no known toxic effects of taking large doses of vitamin B_{12}, but neither is there any scientific evidence that extra vitamin B_{12} helps boost energy. Vitamin B_{12} has no established UL.

231. CHOOSE FOODS RICH IN VITAMIN B₁₂

Foods rich in B_{12} include poultry, milk and other fortified dairy products, clams, liver, beef, oysters, crab, and tuna. Vegetarians may need supplemental vitamins.

232. TAKE FOLIC ACID

Folic acid's main role is to maintain the cell's genetic code—DNA, the master plan for cell reproduction. It also works with vitamin B_{12} to form hemoglobin in red blood cells.

Deficiencies of folic acid include anemia, impaired growth, and abnormal digestive function. Taking too much folic acid through supplements can mask a vitamin B_{12} deficiency and could interfere with other medications. In the synthetic form—the form used to fortify foods and in supplements—folic acid has a UL of 1,000 mcg per day for adults over eighteen.

233. CHOOSE FOODS RICH IN FOLIC ACID

Foods rich in folic acid include some fruits, such as oranges, as well as leafy vegetables, legumes, liver, wheat germ, some fortified cereals, avocados, and enriched-grain products.

234. TAKE BIOTIN

Biotin participates in the metabolism of the macronutrients for energy and helps your body produce energy in the cells. For people who eat a healthy, well-balanced diet, deficiency is not a problem. In the rare cases when deficiency does occur, symptoms include heart abnormalities, loss of appetite, fatigue, depression, and dry skin. Biotin has no known toxic effects and no established UL.

235. CHOOSE FOODS RICH IN BIOTIN

This vitamin is found in a wide variety of foods, such as eggs, liver, yeast breads, cereals, wheat germ, and oatmeal.

236. TAKE PANTOTHENIC ACID

Like biotin, pantothenic acid also participates in the metabolism of the macronutrients for energy and helps your body produce energy in the cells. In addition, pantothenic acid functions in the production of some hormones and neurotransmitters in the brain. When deficiency does occur, symptoms include nausea, fatigue, and difficulty sleeping. The only possible effects of consuming too much pantothenic acid are occasional diarrhea and water retention. Pantothenic acid has no established UL.

237. CHOOSE FOODS RICH IN PANTOTHENIC ACID

Foods rich in pantothenic acid include meat, poultry, fish, whole-grain cereals, legumes, yogurt, sweet potatoes, milk, and eggs.

238. TAKE VITAMIN C (ASCORBIC ACID)

As an antioxidant, vitamin C may reduce the risk of heart disease by preventing the oxidation of LDL (low-density lipoprotein or "bad" cholesterol), which decreases the risk for plaque formation, which can clog arteries and lead to a heart attack or stroke. Vitamin C also protects vitamin E from oxidation. Vitamin C may also prevent blood vessels from constricting and thus cutting off blood supply to the heart. Studies have shown that 1,000 to 2,000 milligrams of vitamin C per day can help block the dangerous artery-destroying effects of the amino acid homocysteine. Supplementing with 500 milligrams of vitamin C per day may lower blood pressure by increasing the activity and levels of nitric oxide, which relaxes arteries and lowers blood pressure. Nitric oxide also helps prevent clot formation and plaque buildup on artery walls. So, load up on C!

239. CHOOSE FOODS RICH IN VITAMIN C

Most fruits and vegetables are great sources of vitamin C. Foods particularly high in C include hot chili peppers (raw), cantaloupe, sweet peppers, dark green leafy vegetables, tomatoes, kiwi fruit, oranges, and mango. You can safely take up to 2,000 milligrams per day, but anything over 2,500 may affect blood or urine tests.

240. DON'T OVERDO VITAMIN C

Because vitamin C is a water-soluble vitamin, your body excretes the excess that may be consumed. Very large doses, though, could cause kidney stones, nausea, and diarrhea. The effects of taking large amounts over extended periods of time are not yet known. Vitamin C has a UL set at 2,000 mg per day for adults over eighteen.

241. CONSIDER RIBOFLAVIN TO COMBAT MIGRAINES

Preliminary research indicates that taking a high dose of riboflavin (400 milligrams) every day may help prevent migraine headaches. Researchers caution that you need to make sure that your headaches are true migraines, and that it works best if you have migraines at least twice a month. For those with diagnosed migraines, supplementing with riboflavin might be worth a try. Most riboflavin supplements contain no more than 100 milligrams per tablet, so you'll need a prescription to get one that contains 400 milligrams. Talk to your doctor before treating your migraines with riboflavin supplements. ✳

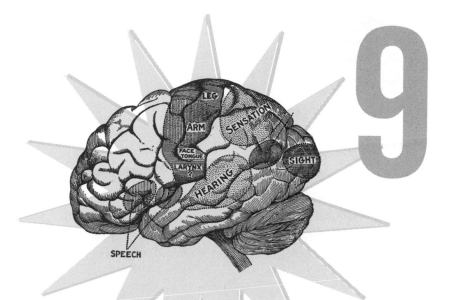

CLEANSE
YOUR
BRAIN

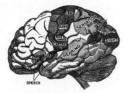

CLEANSE YOUR BRAIN

You can cleanse your brain of harmful toxins.

242. DETOXIFY YOUR BRAIN

If you suspect that you may have been exposed to dangerous fumes or toxic chemicals, consult a doctor for a thorough analysis and treatment. To cleanse your brain (and your body) of common toxins, such as pollutants or household chemicals, you can try: flaxseed, licorice root, ginseng, ginkgo biloba, aloe vera, grapefruit pectin, papayas, slippery elm bark, alfalfa, peppermint, and ginger tea. You can take capsules or use the ingredients to make tea. You can also drink lemon water, exercise strenuously, take a sauna, get a vigorous massage, and eat a high fiber cleansing diet. Deep breathing exercises, in clean environments, will infuse your brain with fresh oxygen. When it comes to minimizing food contaminants, wash all fruits and vegetables thoroughly.

243. DE-STRESS THROUGH EXERCISE

Yoga, Pilates, stretching, and other mind-body exercises relax the mind as well as the body by helping link movement to the breath, which, in turn, stops the physical response to stress. These gentle levels of activity can burn off the physical tension, relax your muscles, and, at the same time, keep your worrying brain from obsessing about a concern for too long. Regular exercise, even if it's begun at a very advanced age, has been shown to help stave off heart disease, type 2 diabetes, and other serious diseases. It also helps maintain brain health and function and maintains, and can even improve, bone density.

244. EXPRESS YOUR EMOTIONS

Feelings and emotions are almost identical in context. However, there are subtle differences. A feeling is a bodily sensation. If you stub your toe, you feel pain. Emotions are involuntary physical responses to events in life. A blush, a laugh, an increased heart rate, a sudden loss of color, or tears are all examples of an emotional reaction. An emotion may be fleeting or it may remain for days, or even years. The ability to feel enables a person to identify an emotion as something that is either positive or negative. It is when an individual represses an undesirable emotion (such as hidden anger, guilt, or self-hatred) that psychological damage can occur. Acknowledging your emotions and working your way through them will free up your brain.

245. DEAL WITH YOUR PHOBIA

A phobia is an unreasonable, compulsive, persistent fear of any specific type of object, animal, insect, or situation. Having to face something that a person fears can produce a phobia anxiety attack. Such an attack may have a number of physical reactions: heart palpitations, breathlessness, weakness, an uncontrollable feeling of terror, and hysterical screaming. Anxiety and phobias are closely related. Stress and unresolved conflicts can lead to a chronic state of anxiety. Individuals suffering from chronic anxiety may develop a phobia as a safety net. As long as they avoid the phobia-producing object, animal, or situation, they can repress their ever-present anxiety and lead a fairly stable life. However, when the person encounters the fear-inducing object, the repressed anxiety may erupt into a phobic panic attack.

246. KNOW THE DANGERS TO YOUR NERVOUS SYSTEM

All systems in the human body are vulnerable to environmental hazards such as toxic chemicals, but the nervous system is at special risk for some very important reasons:

▶ Neurons normally cannot regenerate once they are lost, unlike other types of cells.

▶ Nerve-cell loss and other changes to the nervous system occur progressively during the later years of life. As a result, toxic damage may occur simultaneously with aging.

▶ Many neurotoxic chemicals are easily able to cross the blood-brain barrier, causing damage to sensitive regions of the brain.

▶ Toxic chemicals often interfere with the nervous system's sensitive electrochemical balance, upsetting the balance necessary for the proper communication of information throughout the body.

247. CLEAN UP YOUR ENVIRONMENT

Free radicals are the natural by-products of many processes within and among cells. As we've noted, keeping free radicals under control protects your heart and your brain. Inhalation of toxic dust (such as asbestos, quartz, or silica) can lead to lung injury that is partially mediated by free radical production. In addition, a wide variety of environmental agents including photochemical air pollutants—pesticides, solvents, anesthetics, exhaust fumes, and the general class of aromatic hydrocarbons—also cause free radical damage to cells. Since free radicals are also created by exposure to various external environmental factors such as tobacco smoke and radiation, cleaning up your environment can benefit your brain.

248. USE CAUTION WHEN USING TOXIC CHEMICALS

The skin is our first line of defense in protecting the inside of the body from the outside environment. Skin is tough and offers very good protection from most pollutants, but it's not perfect. Harmful agents can enter the bloodstream if the protective layer of waxy liquid on the skin's surface is broken or dissolved. As a result, it's always a good idea to wear sufficient protection when working with potentially dangerous chemicals, such as cleaning products, pesticides, and solvents.

249. CHECK FOR LEAD EXPOSURE

Lead poses one of the greatest health threats when it gets in our water. In high doses, this metal, which once was commonly used in household plumbing, can cause severe brain damage and even death; in low doses, it can cause nerve system damage in still-developing fetuses, infants, and children. Those most at risk are individuals living in homes constructed between 1910 and 1940, when lead service pipes were commonly used. Also risky are homes with plumbing consisting of copper pipes connected by lead-based solder (which was banned by federal law in 1986) and older chrome-plated bathroom fixtures, which are made of brass consisting of 3 to 8 percent lead. If you suspect your home may be subject to lead contamination, have it tested.

250. CHECK FOR FORMALDEHYDE

Formaldehyde is used in the manufacture of a wide number of household products, including plywood, particle board, paneling, counter tops, flooring, and carpeting. These products often exude formaldehyde in a process known as "outgassing," resulting in chronic respiratory problems in millions of Americans. Those living in newly built tract homes, condominiums, townhouses, and mobile homes risk greater exposure because they tend to use more products known to contain the chemical. If you suffer from unexplained respiratory problems, headaches, or other mysterious symptoms, you could be the victim of formaldehyde exposure. To reduce your risk, air out items known to contain high levels of the chemical, such as new furniture and carpeting, before bringing them into your home.

251. TAKE ACTION

Your first step, of course, should be to identify all potential sources of indoor air pollution, then take the necessary steps to eliminate them. Walk from room to room and note all possible problems, such as badly vented heaters, appliances in poor repair, and a lack of early warning systems, such as carbon monoxide and radon detectors. In addition, make sure you review all lifestyle issues that could adversely affect the air quality in your home, such as tobacco use, the frequent use of chemical cleaning agents and solvents, and even chemicals used in hobbies, such as industrial glue or paint. Every time you use such items without taking proper precautions, such as opening windows for ventilation and using a respirator, you pollute the air you breathe and endanger your health.

252. OPEN YOUR WINDOWS

Make sure your home is well ventilated. Open all the windows whenever possible and consider exhaust fans or air-to-air heat-exchanging devices that draw fresh air in through one duct and expel it through another. In addition, make sure stoves and heaters all vent outdoors. Keeping your house constantly closed tight not only prevents harmful pollutants from dissipating, but also promotes sick building syndrome. ✳

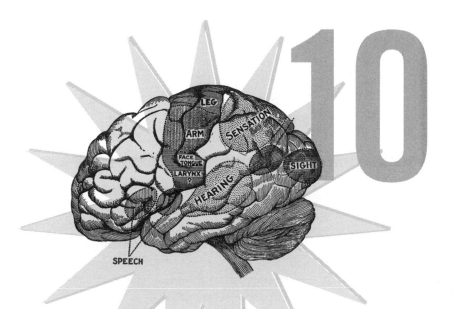

TRAIN
YOUR
BRAIN

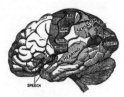

TRAIN YOUR BRAIN

Use the brain's power to your advantage.

253. THINK POSITIVELY

According to Daniel G. Amen, MD, author of *Making a Good Brain Great*, every thought releases brain chemicals. Positive, happy, hopeful, optimistic, joyful thoughts produce yummy chemicals that create a sense of well being and help your brain function at peak capacity; unhappy, miserable, negative, dark thoughts have the opposite effect, effectively slowing down your brain and even creating depression. If you tend to focus on what can go wrong, or what is wrong, or how unhappy you are, or how someone hurt you, these negative thoughts can dim your brain's capacity to function. It saps the brain of its positive forcefulness. Dr. Amen suggests writing out negative thoughts to dispel their power over your brain.

254. USE YOUR IMAGINATION

According to Dr. Frank Lawlis in *The IQ Answer*, "The mechanism in the brain follows the imagery process . . . we only know our world through our senses and our interpretations of those sensations." He notes the power of hypnosis to solicit reactions to stimuli that isn't present, such as someone puckering when told they were sucking a lemon. "If we hold on to the idea of those sensations, our bodies [and brains] do not know the difference. The process is pretty simple. The imagery stimulates the same neurological network as the actual experience." Your prefrontal cortex seeks to create what you think you want. Thus, envisioning exactly what you want, or simply envisioning positive outcomes, and keeping it in the forefront of your mind helps you create the desired outcome.

255. TURN IT ON
According to Daniel G. Amen, MD, author of *Making a Good Brain Great*, placebos (an inert substance with no physiological effects, i.e., no medicinal properties) are astonishingly effective. He noted that 150 years ago, doctors relied more on their relationship with their patients and the administration of placebos to treat illnesses. Apparently many patients improved based on how much they trusted their doctor and how much they believed that they would get well. Recent studies have found that issuing placebos to reduce pain can be one-half to two-thirds as powerful as morphine. If patients believe that the placebo is a pain reliever, it causes physiological changes in their brain that reduces their pain.

256. TAME YOUR EMOTIONS
So-called type A people, with a tough, aggressive, hard-driving style, are at risk for heart disease. Now, however, it is being recognized, according to a study by psychologist Tilmer Engebretson at Ohio State University in Columbus, that people who have a trait he names "cynical hostility" are at greater risk for developing heart-tissue damage than are their nonhostile colleagues. Other reports have shown a connection between hostility in healthy people and the subsequent development of atherosclerosis and high cholesterol. One study at Duke University showed that cynicism, mistrust, and aggressive anger increased the death rate

from heart disease. If you struggle with these feelings, find a therapist, attend a support group, write it out, deal with it, and eradicate it. Focus on positive emotions and train your brain to experience more soothing emotions.

257. SEE A THERAPIST

Therapy is designed to alter the way you perceive your life and the challenges it presents. A good therapist helps you put things in perspective, tame emotional mood swings, and reframe problems. As you learn to reframe, your behavior generally follows. Having positive thoughts and taking positive action bolsters positive brain pathways and thus ultimately leads to improved brain function. Several studies have shown that cognitive therapy, i.e., talk therapy that teaches patients to counter negative thought patterns by replacing them with positive thoughts, has enhanced brain function.

258. CURB ANY WORRYWART TENDENCIES

It is well known that a long continued fear or worry will deplete an individual's vitality; it will cause him to feel out of sorts, below par, or not himself. Under these conditions the body loses its natural resistance to disease. It is in a fit state to become the prey of any infection and any form of illness. Excessive, habitual worrying also keeps your brain running around in circles, often in flight-or-fight mode, which taxes your entire body—particularly your brain. You can train your brain to think positively and, with enough redirection of the internal dialogue, you can improve your health, your outlook on life, your energy, and your brain.

259. EXPRESS GRATITUDE

Focus on what you love about your life and your emotional brain fires up. You are more coordinated. Write out five things you're grateful for today. Focus on what is making you feel lucky and good about your life. This trains your brain to focus on the love and pleasant experiences in your life. Do it long enough and you'll effectively create a positive groove in your brain that will create ripple effects in your life. ✹

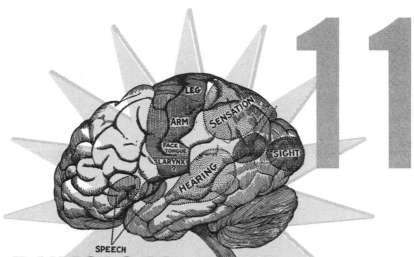

PHYSICAL
EXERCISE TO
BENEFIT
YOUR BRAIN

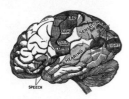

PHYSICAL EXERCISE TO BENEFIT YOUR BRAIN

Use it
or lose it!

260. EXERCISE TO STAY YOUNG

Regular physical activity keeps our muscles toned and strong, helps us maintain our ideal weight by burning calories, maintains bone strength and density, and improves and maintains heart and lung function. Exercise also builds stamina, improves flexibility, boosts our immune system, makes sex more fun, reduces our risk of cancer, improves our reflexes, lowers stress, and benefits our overall physical and mental health. In addition, exercise helps keep our metabolism functioning at maximum capacity, which becomes increasingly important as we age and find it increasingly difficult to process fatty acids. This, in turn, affects almost all of the body's systems, diminishing immune response and increasing our risk of atherosclerotic disease. Simply taking a thirty-minute walk every day can reduce your risk of heart attack after just five months, doctors report.

261. STAY MENTALLY AND PHYSICALLY ACTIVE

In 2005, Ohio State University researchers reported that older people who exercised regularly were more likely to maintain the mental acuity they needed to do everyday tasks like follow a recipe and keep track of the pills they take. Some of the recommended mental activities for older people included crossword puzzles, trivia games, Scrabble, card games, and projects, such as fixing appliances and cooking. A study published in the *Proceedings of the National Academy of Science (PNAS)* in 2001 investigated the benefits of keeping active both mentally and physically during leisure time to prevent Alzheimer's. A group of inactive adults between twenty and sixty years of age was compared to more active peers. Researchers took into account all variables and still found that the risk of developing Alzheimer's in inactive people was four times that of active people.

262. MOVE YOUR BODY

According to author David Rakel, in his 2002 book *Integrative Medicine*, over 10,000 trials have examined the relationship between exercise and mood, showing that exercise may be just as effective in treating depression as psychotherapy. Exercise stimulates circulation and increases blood flow to all parts of the body and brain, bringing extra oxygen, glucose, and nutrients. Exercise increases self-esteem and confidence, which makes you stand up straighter and look the rest of the world squarely in the eye. In animal studies, exercise helps increase healthy growth factors in the memory center of the brain. It doesn't even matter what kind of exercise you choose. You can walk, jog, swim, lift weights, do yoga or tai chi—it all works.

263. START SLOWLY

If you haven't been active for a long time, or particularly if you are elderly and generally inactive, start slow. Even if you start sitting in a chair and doing stretches, that can help. Then you can hold 2-pound weights and flex your arms. After a while, you can graduate to 5-pound weights. For your hips and legs, just start by getting in and out of a chair about ten times. Slowly but surely, you can build up those weak muscles that are crying out for exercise.

264. TAKE A BRISK WALK

Physical exercise helps us lose excess weight, increase our physical strength, and reduce stress. Physical exercise increases the blood flow to the brain, bringing oxygen and nutrients and taking away waste products. Brisk walking for thirty minutes a day is all that is needed for brain health.

265. EXERCISE 30 MINUTES A DAY

Regular exercise—at least twenty minutes a day, but thirty minutes to an hour daily is best—is one great way to preserve your mental acuity. Aerobic exercise helps get the blood coursing through your system, carrying oxygen and glucose to your brain—two substances the brain needs in order to function. Regular exercise also can prod the brain into producing more molecules that help protect and produce the brain's neurons. Though studies are still underway to establish the link between exercise and increased brain neurons, many researchers—including those involved with Alzheimer's disease research—are studying the protective effects of regular physical exercise on the brain's neural paths for transmitting signals. Exercise has a lot of connotations, but exercise can mean walking around the neighborhood. What's important is that you do something that requires some physicality, limbers up your muscles, and improves your circulation. The U.S. federal guidelines for exercise say that getting at least thirty minutes a day most days a week will help prevent heart disease, osteoporosis, diabetes, obesity, and now, perhaps, Alzheimer's.

266. INCREASE ACTIVITY

Exercises that increase stamina greatly benefit the heart and lungs. These activities involve far more exertion than general physical activity and include such things as running, cycling, swimming, tennis, and racquetball. The goal is to strengthen the heart and lungs by working both at full capacity. If you haven't exercised in a while, it's a good idea to start slowly and gradually increase the amount of exercise you do in a week. As your stamina increases, you'll find it easier to do more and more. If you're over forty, it's also wise to get a physical exam from your doctor before starting any type of stamina-building exercise—just to be on the safe side.

267. LIFT WEIGHTS

Exercises to increase strength and flexibility include weight lifting (whether through the use of free weights or the kind of weight machines found in most gyms), yoga, and similar stretching activities. Weight-bearing exercises are particularly important for women because they can help prevent the onset of osteoporosis later in life by maintaining bone density before, during, and after menopause. And you don't have to lift weights until you bulge like Mr. Universe; most health specialists say thirty to forty minutes of weight training a week is sufficient to maintain optimum health. Weight training can vastly improve muscle strength, balance, and flexibility—all of which is good for your brain.

268. DON'T OVERDO IT

A study of male Harvard graduates compared longevity rates of major athletes (meaning those who lettered in a particular sport), minor athletes (those who participated but didn't letter), and nonathletes. It was assumed that the major athletes, who presumably exercised the hardest, would have the greatest longevity, but, in fact, it was the minor athletes who lived the longest.

What does this mean? Well, for starters, it means that when it comes to life-extending physical activity, moderation is best. There's no need to train like an Olympic athlete, because too much exercise is just as bad as too little. The key is to strengthen and maintain your body's systems, not abuse them, which is what an excessive physical regimen does. If you feel pain, you may be working too hard. Slow down and listen to your body. It will tell you what it needs and when you've gone too far.

269. ALTERNATE WORKOUTS

A well-rounded exercise regimen should strengthen muscles, benefit the heart and lungs, and build endurance. For optimum results, alternate weight training, aerobics, and circuit training. Reliance on only one form of exercise will not benefit your entire body. *Vary your activities to ensure a complete workout.* Weight lifting strengthens your muscles and may help you lose that dangerous belly fat; you'll also need some cardiovascular activity, such as aerobics, to benefit your heart and lungs—and thus your circulatory system and blood flow to your brain.

270. HIRE A PERSONAL TRAINER

Or at least consult a personal trainer. If you have trouble staying motivated, a personal trainer can be extremely beneficial. In addition to making sure you exercise regularly, he or she can show you how to perform your workout for maximum advantage. Most gyms have staff that will create the exercise regimen that's best for you and help you through it. This ensures that you are exercising correctly and at the proper pace. If you can afford a personal trainer, he or she will encourage you to commit to your routine and to push yourself just a wee bit harder—all of which is good for your brain.

271. JOIN A TEAM
Many are turned off by the regimented workout available at a fitness center. If you prefer company with your activity, consider joining a baseball, softball, tennis, bowling, or racquetball league. All of these activities benefit the heart, lungs, muscles—and your brain!

272. PLAY TABLE TENNIS
Daniel G. Amen, MD, author of *Making a Good Brain Great*, is a major enthusiast of table tennis, calling it "the best brain sport ever": "It is highly aerobic, uses both the upper and lower body, is great for hand-eye coordination and reflexes, and causes you to use many different areas of the brain at once as you are tracking the ball, planning shots and strategies, and figuring out spins. It is like aerobic chess." He also noted that it is the second most popular organized sport in the world, and has been an Olympic sport since 1988.

273. SHAKE IT UP
Consider some fun alternatives to the traditional exercise activities, such as calisthenics, dance aerobics, water exercise, bicycling, Pilates, and yoga. Take a country line or ballroom dancing class, or join a mountain-biking, birdwatching, hiking, or dog-walking club. It's important that you enjoy your exercise regimen, because it reduces the chances that you'll get bored and quit.

274. PRACTICE PILATES

By emphasizing the importance of the mind/body connection in attaining physical fitness, Joseph Pilates married critical elements of Eastern and Western philosophies. Westerners approach health and fitness as a scientific function of maintaining and nurturing the body's muscles, bones, and circulatory and digestive systems. Eastern philosophies place much more importance on the development of mental and spiritual powers in the pursuit of pure health. Pilates students approach each movement with focus and determination, and they engage body and mind equally in each physical endeavor. Pilates is a conditioning program designed to work the whole body—including your brain—simultaneously and uniformly. Joseph Pilates created his exercises with the intention "that each muscle may cooperatively and loyally aid in the uniform development of all our muscles. Developing minor muscles naturally helps to strengthen major muscles." As a result, every muscle is developed in every movement.

275. PRACTICE YOGA

Yoga is an ancient Indian method of exercise designed to "yoke" body and mind that involves specific postures, breathing exercise, and meditation. It provides an excellent fitness activity on its own and also makes the perfect complement to other fitness activities because it increases strength, flexibility, circulation, posture, and overall body condition. Practicing yoga is great both for people who have a hard time slowing down (you'll learn how great it feels and how important it is to move your body with slow control) and for people who have a hard time engaging in high-impact or fast-paced exercise. You can adapt your routine to your own fitness level to make it decidedly low impact, and among the more perfect stress management exercises. Its original purpose was to gain control over the body and bring it into a state of balance in order to free the mind for spiritual contemplation. Yoga can help you to master your body so that it doesn't master you.

276. PRACTICE TAI CHI

Although tai chi is technically an ancient Chinese martial art, there is nothing martial about it, although it is still artistic. Tai chi is made up of a series of flowing, slow movements that are connected with the breath. The individual movements are called *forms*, and each form often recalls an animal or something in nature, such as a tree or reed. Some form names include "Grasp the bird's tail" and "Wave hands like clouds." These names are evocative of the movement, which incorporate all the limbs and the breath. Research on tai chi has found it to be helpful for mood disorders, such as anxiety and depression, as well as physical ailments, such arthritis and hypertension (high blood pressure). Because you perform tai chi while standing and use your whole body, it can build muscular strength and slightly increase cardiovascular function. More than anything, though, tai chi is great for balance training, flexibility, and relaxation—and thus excellent for your brain.

277. BE LIKE JACK

Jack LaLanne opened the first commercial health club in Oakland, California, in 1936. LaLanne's astounding physical feats have generated a lot of publicity over the years. Among the most remarkable are the following:

► At age 61, LaLanne celebrated the nation's bicentennial by swimming the length of Long Beach Harbor (about 1 mile) while handcuffed, shackled, and towing thirteen boats (one for each of the original thirteen colonies).

- On his seventieth birthday, LaLanne braved strong currents and blustery winds to tow seventy boats and seventy people a total of 1.5 miles—again while handcuffed and shackled.

What's the secret to LaLanne's astounding physical endurance? He maintains a rigorous devotion to proper nutrition and rigorous exercise. He consumes about 450 vitamin and mineral supplements daily and eats nothing but natural foods. His diet is rich in fruits and vegetables, and he avoids red meat, substituting poultry instead. He also avoids dietary fat. His exercise regimen is just as demanding. He works out two and a half hours each day, combining weight training with aerobic exercise for endurance. Okay, don't go overboard, but let Jack inspire you to eat a healthy diet and exercise. ✳

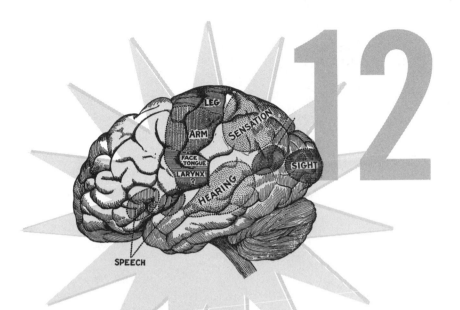

SOOTHE
YOUR
BRAIN

153

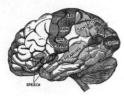

SOOTHE YOUR BRAIN

Tune out the stress to recharge your brain.

278. TURN DOWN THE NOISE

The most striking area in which older people and younger people differ is in how they remember. In general, younger people are more adept at learning and retaining information in the face of distractions such as television, loud music, or crowds. Their brains, it seems, are better at multitasking, that is, engaging in several functions at once, such as watching a movie on TV while cramming for a history exam. Older people, as a rule, require a quieter environment in which to digest new information for later retrieval. Studies have concluded that this dramatic generational difference in learning and memorizing is due to the fact that older people have greater difficulty filtering out useless stimuli, such as music or conversation. Their brains absorb everything, affecting the memorization of pertinent information. For this reason, seniors are encouraged to read or study in a quiet environment, where they won't be easily distracted and can focus on the task at hand. Silence can be not only therapeutic but also remarkably energizing. Finding a space each day for silence and stillness allows the body to recharge.

279. WATCH A FUNNY MOVIE

Laugh! It really is the best medicine—for both our minds and our bodies. For one thing, a good sense of humor provides needed stress relief. When we laugh at our problems rather than fret over them, they become less serious and thus easier to solve. Humor also improves cognitive function by keeping the mind active and encouraging creative thinking—a vital defense against age—and provides an important emotional catharsis during periods of emotional tension. Researchers at Loma Linda University School of Medicine's Department of Clinical Immunology conducted numerous studies proving that laughter helps lower serum cortisol levels, increases the amount of activated T lymphocytes, increases the number and activity of natural killer cells, and increases the number of T cells that have helper/suppressor receptors. In other words, laughter helps stimulate the immune system and counters the immunosuppressive effects of stress. Laughter also benefits the heart, improves oxygen flow to the brain, and works the muscles in the head, neck, chest, and pelvis—in much the same way as the stress reduction exercises of yoga. This helps keep muscles loose and limber and enables them to rest more easily. So rent a funny movie, go to a comedy club, or watch a comedy show and laugh!

280. ADOPT A PET

One of the most consistent findings among the many studies evaluating the beneficial role of pets in our lives is that they provide an important measure of stress relief. Simply petting or playing with our favorite pet, whether it's a dog, cat, hamster, or canary, stimulates the production of calming chemicals within the brain and helps us relax. Watching fish in an aquarium has a similar calming effect. The calming influence of small animals is so effective that many doctors recommend daily pet play as therapy for their patients who are under a lot of stress either at work or at home. Fifteen minutes of tossing a yarn ball to some frolicsome kittens is a wonderful and inexpensive way to shed the stress of a hard day at the office. If you're not a cat person, playing fetch with your dog is equally beneficial. The point is to spend time with your pet, whatever the species, and enjoy its company. Talk to it. Pet it. Scratch it behind the ears. Bask in the glow of the pet-owner bond and feel the anxiety melt away. Even the most stressful day is no match for a puppy that's so happy to see you that its tail is a blur.

281. TAKE A VACATION

Sometimes our environment is the biggest stressor in our lives. If it's been a while since you've taken a vacation, get as far away from the source of your troubles as you can and enjoy yourself. If money is a worry, make it a low-cost holiday, perhaps one of those vacations where you volunteer to build a house or teach a class. Most importantly, don't take your problems with you! Leave work at the office and home problems at the front door. Give your brain, your body, and your soul a vacation.

282. CURB YOUR STRESS

Reduce the amount of stress and anxiety in your life. Stress is one of the most common causes of transient insomnia; it keeps the brain awake and functioning long into the night or wee hours of the morning. Stress causes worry, and worry interferes with sleep. Acknowledging the problem is the first step, followed by a resolution to take care of those problems you can and a promise not to dwell on those you can't. Excessive stress creates tension and anxiety and can lead to a variety of health problems that are not obviously linked to tension. Stress can also complicate pre-existing conditions.

These are the key symptoms:

- ▶ Inability to relax
- ▶ Emotional instability/mood swings
- ▶ Headaches
- ▶ Sleeplessness

283. RELIEVE YOUR STRESS

An October 2000 *Brain Research Bulletin* study confirmed what has been known since the mid-1980s: Cortisol levels are high in Alzheimer's patients. This study also showed that high levels of cortisol correlated with a more rapid deterioration of the Mini-Mental State Examination (a 30-point questionnaire used to screen for dementia) over a forty-month period in a group of elderly women. It is well known that chronic stress elevates cortisol levels, which is one of the main causes of brain cell death. Popular stress reduction techniques include regular prayer, meditation, and self-hypnosis.

284. FIX IT OR FORGET IT

Do what you can to resolve the stressful situations in your life and stop worrying about those you can't resolve. After all, what's the sense of losing sleep and harming your health dwelling on things over which you have no control? There's no point in mulling things over endlessly in your mind. Free your brain; fix it or forget it.

285. LIGHT AN AROMATIC CANDLE

Smell is the most potent of all the senses because the information is delivered straight to your hypothalymus. As moods, motivation, and creativity all stem from the hypothalymus, odors affect all of these processes. Think of a disgusting odor and how it can affect your appetite—or think of a fragrance that brings back a pleasant memory of a loved one, and you'll get the idea of how intimately intertwined scents are with our emotions, memories, and ideas. Light a candle whose fragrance invokes pleasant memories, lie back, and soothe your hypothalymus.

286. HAVE A CUP OF CHAMOMILE TEA

Chamomile tea is widely known for its relaxing properties as well as its apple-like aroma, and is known to soothe the nerves and restore vitality. Contemporary herbalists also recommend chamomile for fever, digestive upsets, anxiety, and insomnia. British researchers recently discovered that chamomile stimulates the immune system's white blood cells. It's particularly recommended for use at the onset of a cold or the flu and its warming and soothing properties promote sleep, the greatest curative of all. Drink a cup or two of tea for relaxation, or at night to promote sleep. **Caution:** Generally speaking, chamomile is one of the safest herbs available. However, if you are allergic to ragweed or have ever suffered anaphylactic shock, avoid this herb.

287. TRY HOPS

A thousand years ago brewers of English ale began using hops as a preservative. Much later they added it as an ingredient and discovered that their pickers suffered two peculiar effects: They tired quickly when working and the female pickers got their menstrual periods earlier than normal. Science has since recognized the remarkable power of hops as a sedative. It has a calming effect on the body, soothes muscle spasms, relieves nervous tension, and promotes restful sleep. If you suffer from insomnia, make a tea with 1 teaspoon of dried hops in a cup of boiling water and drink it at bedtime. Capsules are also available. Externally, an old-fashioned cure for sleeplessness is to sleep on a small pillowcase filled with hops sprinkled with alcohol.

288. TRY VALERIAN INSTEAD OF VALIUM

Called "the Valium of the nineteenth century" (though it has no chemical similarity to Valium), the herb valerian (*Valeriana officinalis*) is a common sedative used worldwide. In Europe, it is prescribed for anxiety. Herbalists have chosen valerian for treatment of nervous tension and even for panic attacks. It is known as a safe non-narcotic herbal sedative and is often combined with other herbs to make pain-relieving remedies, as it has the ability to relax muscle spasms. Despite the fact that valerian has been widely studied, just how it works remains a mystery.

289. TRY SNAKEROOT

For centuries, the plant Indian snakeroot was used in Ayurvedic medicine for a range of problems, including anxiety, headache, fevers, and snakebites. Mahatma Gandhi was reputed to drink a cup of snakeroot tea at bedtime if he had had a busy day and felt overstimulated. Western herbalists valued it as a powerful tranquilizer and also used it to treat high blood pressure.

Then, in 1947, scientists at the CIBA company extracted the alkaloid reserpine from snakeroot and began marketing a drug called Serpasil for high blood pressure. This drug proved to have many unpleasant side effects, and in the 1950s, a new tranquilizer was developed from the herb. This has always been a prescription-only drug in the United States, but in other parts of the world, including Europe and Asia, snakeroot in its natural state continues to be widely used as a soothing tea and tranquilizer.

290. RELAX WITH DARK CHOCOLATE

Two researchers at the Neurosciences Institute in San Diego, California, Daniel Piomelli and Emmanuelle diTomaso, discovered in a 1996 study that chocolate contains a pharmacologically active substance that has the same effect on the brain as marijuana, and that this chemical may be responsible for certain drug-induced psychoses associated with chocolate craving. The chemical in question is a neurotransmitter known as anandamide which is produced naturally in the brain, and is also a component of chocolate. This finding should not imply that eating chocolate will get you high; however, this particular compound (and there may be more) provides that "good feeling" you get from eating quality chocolate.

291. CONSIDER ESSENTIAL OILS

Today, people all over the world are paying attention to the healing effects of essential oils, and scientists are continuing to conduct research in an attempt to understand more about the effects of these amazing aromas on the human mind, body, and psychology. Essential oils are extracted from the aromatic essences of certain plants, trees, fruits, flowers, herbs, and spices. Natural volatile oils, they have identifiable chemical and medicinal properties. At this point, over 150 have been extracted, and each has its own definitive scent and unique healing properties. For optimum benefit, the oils must be extracted from natural raw ingredients, with attention to purity. They must be stored in dark, tightly stoppered glass bottles and kept away from light and heat in order to maintain their potency. They can be used individually or in combination.

292. LEARN ABOUT ESSENTIAL OILS

Essential oils and their actions are extremely complex. In addition to being antiseptic, each also possesses individual properties. The collective qualities of each give it a dominant characteristic, whether it be stimulating, calming, energizing, or relaxing. Essential oils have psychological effects, and they also have notable physiological effects, which means that within the body, they are able to operate in three ways: pharmacologically, physiologically, and psychologically. From the pharmacological perspective, the oils react with body chemistry similarly to drugs, but with a slower and more sympathetic effect and with fewer side effects. In addition, certain oils have a particular affinity for different body parts—spice oils, for example, tend to benefit the digestive system. Some oils, like lavender, are known as adaptogens, which as the name implies, adapt to whatever condition needs assistance. The psychological effect is triggered by the connection the aromatic molecules make with the brain.

293. SAMPLE ESSENTIAL OILS

There are a large number of relaxing aromatic oils on the market, but the best include lavender, sage, sandalwood, frankincense, and chamomile. How you use them is up to you. Some people light scented candles as they relax after a hard day's work or place fragrant potpourri throughout their home. Others prefer to place a few drops of scented oils in their water while they relax in a hot bath or a few drops of scented oil on their pillow to help them unwind and fall asleep faster at night. The important thing is to select a fragrance that is both appealing and relaxing. Floral scents tend to work best, because food scents can make us hungry. Avoid tart or biting fragrances, such as lemon, because they may have the opposite effect, perking you up instead of calming you down. You may have to experiment until you find the scent that is right for you, but it's well worth the effort.

294. USE CAUTION WHEN . . .

Although aromatherapy is compatible with herbal remedies and conventional medicine, it should not be used under the following conditions without the consultation of a qualified practitioner:

- ► If you are pregnant
- ► If you have allergies
- ► If you have a chronic medical condition such as high blood pressure or epilepsy
- ► If you are receiving medical or psychiatric treatment
- ► If you are taking homeopathic remedies
- ► If you have any chronic or serious health problem such as a heart condition

However, aromatherapy is safe to use at home for minor or short-term problems, such as mild depression, tension, or minor ills, so long as you follow safety guidelines:

- ► Do not take essential oils internally.
- ► Do not put essential oils in the eyes.
- ► Do not use essential oils to treat young children.
- ► Keep all oils away from children.
- ► Do not apply undiluted oils directly to the skin.

Anyone wanting to use essential oils can avail himself or herself of a wealth of additional information for every need quite easily. One good Internet source is *www.aromaweb.com.*

295. TAKE A LAVENDER BATH

A warm, lavender-scented bath is a great way to relax and unwind. It also promotes restful sleep. Lavender oil in a hot bath before bed and lavender oil on the pillow can be very relaxing.

296. TRY SAGE AND LEMON BALM EXTRACT

Professor Elaine Perry, of the University of Newcastle upon Tyne in northern England, told members of a medical conference on the psychiatry of old age held in February 2004 that the plant extracts of sage and lemon balm produced promising results in studies to improve memory and behavior in Alzheimer's patients. Dr. Perry said: "In controlled trials in normal volunteers, both extracts improved memory, and lemon balm improved mood. Lemon balm reduced agitation and improved quality of life in people with Alzheimer's disease." ✳

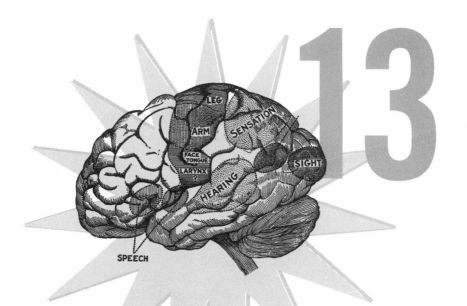

NURTURE
YOUR
BRAIN

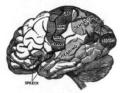

NURTURE YOUR BRAIN

Enrich your life to keep your brain vital.

297. BE AWARE OF YOUR BREATHING

Breath is life. Unfortunately, most adults are shallow breathers. They sip the air the way a Victorian lady sipped her cup of tea, and for the same reason—not to appear coarse. Taking in generous amounts of air seems impolite to many people, especially those who feel socially restricted and insecure about how others will view them. However, breath, like food, nourishes our every cell and cleanses our blood. But, like anorexics, we insist on starving ourselves of this vital nutrient. The good news is that changing breathing patterns is easy. Anyone can do it. Changing your breathing starts with becoming aware of it.

298. PRACTICE BREATHING

Relax and close your eyes. Tell yourself that you are now going to add vital energy every time you inhale deeply. Think of it as putting extra dollars into your energy bank for use whenever you need it. Realize that this vital healing force always surrounds you, that it sustains and nourishes you all the time, even when you are unaware of it. Begin to breathe slowly and rhythmically, not altering your breath pattern but simply becoming aware of it. Now, begin to breathe deeply—slowly and deeply. As you inhale each breath, be aware of the energy coming into your body. Imagine it filling up all the cells of your body like you would fill a balloon by blowing air into it. Let the sense of being filled with energy spread throughout your body. Feel it energize your mind. Hold each breath for a few seconds while you imagine these results. Then, as you exhale feel the energy being retained within you. Let the breath go out smoothly and easily. Do not force or strain.

299. BREATHE FROM YOUR DIAPHRAGM

Abdominal, or diaphragmatic, breathing is "belly" breathing. When the air is taken in, the diaphragm contracts and the abdomen expands; when the air is exhaled, the reverse occurs. You can test yourself for abdominal breathing by laying your hand on your belly as you breathe. If it expands as you inhale, you are breathing with the diaphragm. If it flattens, you are breathing with the chest. To practice abdominal breathing, imagine that your in-breath is filling a balloon in your belly. When the balloon is full, exhale until you feel it is completely empty. Just a few of these deep abdominal breaths will bring relief from tension—and pain is half tension.

300. BREATHE TO RELAX

Sit or lie down in a safe and comfortable spot with no distractions. Loosen any tight clothing; unbutton or untie anything that is restrictive on your body. Begin to breathe *consciously*, following your breath in and out of your lungs. Breathe in through the nostrils, out through the mouth. Pay full attention to your breath, in and out, in and out. Listen to the sound and feel the rhythmic pulsing of it. Continue this until you begin to feel calm and relaxed, a state usually signaled by the breath becoming slow and even.

301. BREATHE TO GATHER POSITIVE ENERGY

You can deepen your relaxation using breath by imagining that you are breathing in *prana*, or the positive vital force of life, and exhaling all tension and negative feeling or experience. One way to do this is to choose two colors, one for the prana and one for the negative energy: See a stream of one color (positive) coming into your body as you inhale, and a stream of the other color (negative) flowing out of your body as you exhale. The colors white and black are easy to identify—white is the pure energy of light, and black represents any dark thoughts. But feel free to use any color that represents healing energy and release of negative energy to you. Don't worry if distracting thoughts arise. Let them float off (you can tell them you will attend to their needs later) like soap bubbles in the air and return to attending to your breathing.

302. LEARN TO MEDITATE

In the late 1960s, Harvard cardiologist Herbert Benson, MD, discovered that relaxation methods caused both psychological and physiological changes that served to counterbalance the body's response to "fight or flight." He called this the "relaxation response." Benson's tests showed that persons who simply sat quietly with their minds focused on a single word, idea, or thought could markedly change their physiology, decreasing metabolism, slowing heart and respiratory rates, and exhibiting brain waves of the alpha-theta pattern. Benson showed that the relaxation response, no matter how it was achieved, caused bodily transformations: Heart rate, breathing rate, muscle tension, and oxygen consumption fall below resting levels; blood pressure can decrease; and the waking brain shifts into the slower patterns associated with reverie and daydreaming. These slightly altered states of consciousness promote healing in the same way sleep does. Meditation also works to train the mind to avoid negative patterns and thought processes, vicious circles of failure, low self-esteem, and even the perception of chronic pain as an intensely negative experience. The brain is a complex and amazing organ, and meditation can teach you to harness your mind's power, integrate your mind and body, and feed your hungry spirit. Meditation comes in many forms, including sitting meditation, walking meditation, mindfulness meditation, yoga meditation, mantra meditation, mandala meditation, visualization, and even prayer.

303. MEDITATE TO STIMULATE

For eons, experts believed meditation calmed the brain, and it does, but it also activates the most thoughtful part of your brain. When you're contemplating serious matters, take time to meditate and you may find yourself making smarter decisions. How does meditation help the mind and body? Studies have found that effective meditation actually increases blood flow to the brain and balances brain wave patterns. It also boosts the immune system and improves cognitive function, including memory.

304. MEDIATE TO RELAX

Here is a "mindless" meditation devised to put you into a state of mind that can lead to real rest. To do this meditation—which is really not a meditation at all in any formal sense—recline or lie down comfortably when you can be alone and uninterrupted for an hour. Turn lights down or off and eliminate outside noises and distractions. Close your eyes and let yourself experience the silence around you, then move inward and find a place of silence inside. Let yourself stay in this place as long as you feel comfortable. Begin to follow your breath without trying to alter it. Just feel the quiet rhythm of your SELF. As you do this, let your mind wander wherever it wants to go, like a puppy let outside for an airing. Follow it if you wish, see what interests it, but make no judgments. Think of your mind as a butterfly lighting on one flower, now on another, gathering nectar. Don't push or move your mind in any particular direction. *Let it go where it wants.* That is the key here. So much meditation tries to harness the mind, tether it like a goat on a rope as bait for large game. Don't do that. As your mind is given the freedom to roam here and there, to *play* at will, it will lead you to your place of rest.

305. GO TO CHURCH

Heart surgery patients who said they received strength and comfort from their religion were three times more likely to survive than those who did not, report researchers at the Dartmouth-Hitchcock Medical Center in Lebanon, New Hampshire. A study of 113 women at the University of North Carolina in Greensboro found a strong link between lower blood pressure and strong religious beliefs— even after factoring in such things as weight, diet, and other lifestyle issues. A study of nearly 92,000 men and women by researchers at Johns Hopkins University in Baltimore found that weekly church-goers died 50 percent less often from heart disease, emphysema, and suicide, and 74 percent less often from cirrhosis, than people who did not attend church.

306. JOIN A SOCIAL CLUB

According to researchers, the more people participate in close social relationships, the better their overall physical and mental health, and the higher their level of function. The definition of *social relationship* is broad and can include everything from daily phone chats with family to regular visits with close friends to attending church every Sunday. The MacArthur Foundation Study on Aging revealed that the two strongest predictors of well-being among the elderly are frequency of visits with friends and frequency of attendance at organization meetings. And the more

meaningful the contribution in a particular activity, the greater the health ber
And it doesn't always have to be people who believe what you believe. Stud
show that the more diverse our innermost circle of social support, the better o.
we are.

307. MAKE FRIENDS

A life rich with friends and loved ones can be one of the best elixirs when it comes to keeping our brains strong and vital. The importance of social support was demonstrated during a recent study at a large nursing home. Residents were randomly divided into three groups and given the task of completing a jigsaw puzzle. All were given four twenty-minute practice sessions, followed by a timed session. Members of the first group were given a lot of verbal encouragement by the experiment director during the practice sessions, members in the second group were given direct assistance, and members of the third group received neither encouragement nor assistance. Those in the group that received a lot of encouragement demonstrated marked improvement in both speed and proficiency in putting the puzzle together during the timed session. In other words, their mental acuity apparently improved. Those who were directly assisted did less well, and those who were left alone showed no change at all. This demonstrates how social support in the form of interaction and encouragement can improve cognitive function in older people. However, it also demonstrates that the support must be appropriate to the individual and what he or she wishes to accomplish, whether it's a stronger memory or improved visual-spatial skills. Daily chats about the previous night's television shows may be seen as social support, but mere conversation with friends won't improve mental tasks. Find supportive friends.

. HOST DINNER PARTIES

nner parties offer great opportunities to socialize and to discuss a wide range
f topics in depth. Invite friends and acquaintances from all walks of life and play
your part as host or hostess by encouraging stimulating conversation. Bone up on
your guests' professions and be ready to introduce controversial or exciting topics
that will engage your mind—and those of your guests. Your guests and your brain
will thank you for it.

309. ATTEND LECTURES

Lectures offer incredible opportunities to learn, to acquire new interests, stay
current, and improve your conversational skills. Pick topics that you know nothing
about—like neuroscience, archeology, quantum physics, ancient history, hiero-
glyphics, etc.—and charge up your brain cells by straining to understand. The
more complex the subject matter, the more it generates new thoughts and gets
your brainwaves sparking.

310. VOLUNTEER

Studies have shown that people who regularly volunteer their time and services
to those in need demonstrate better health and greater longevity than those
who don't. Helping others improves our mood, reduces the effects of stress, and
boosts our immune system. But in order to enjoy the healthful benefits of volun-
teerism, you actually have to participate. Simply writing a check to your favorite charity isn't enough; you need to get out there and become physically—and
mentally—involved. ✳

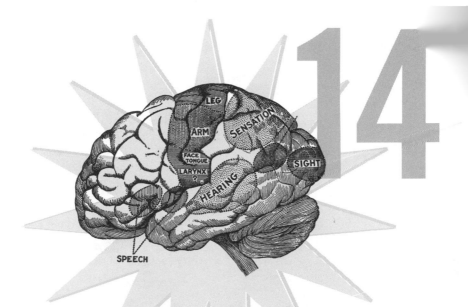

REJUVENATE
YOUR
BRAIN

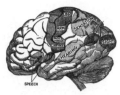

REJUVENATE YOUR BRAIN

Stimulate your brain to keep it young.

311. BELIEVE IN ANTI-AGING POSSIBILITIES

The last few decades have shed tremendous light on how age affects the brain and how we can keep our mental faculties sharp regardless of the number of years under our belts. Senility is not a forgone conclusion for anyone; many common types of mental degeneration are the result of lifestyle more than age and very often can be reversed with a simple change in diet or medication. Believe in the possibility and take proactive steps to keep your brain young.

312. DON'T BE A GEEZER

Today, of course, we know that the stereotypical "demented old geezer" is more myth than medical fact. Old age doesn't automatically mean a substantial loss of memory or other cognitive skills any more than it automatically means heart disease, cancer, or any other supposedly age-related medical condition. Numerous studies have concluded that mental acuity can remain strong even at the 100-year mark and offer as proof the tens of thousands of Americans who have stayed bright and sharp-witted well into their senior years. While many people do develop some form of senility in their later years, far more live out their lives with their mental faculties strong and intact. Mental acuity in our senior years is strongly dependent on regular stimulation, so it's important that you give your mind a mental workout every day.

313. STAY MENTALLY ALERT

The brain is affected by age. Researchers note that the brain tends to shrink an average of 6 percent over our lifetime, resulting in a loss of cognitive abilities such as memory, problem solving, and digesting information. Forgetfulness is, without question, one of the most common "complaints" of aging, though it's more often due to reduced oxygen or a lack of use than to Alzheimer's disease or other organic disorders. Indeed, the phrase "use it or lose it" really applies to the brain; studies have found that older individuals who enjoy solving puzzles, read a lot, or regularly engage in other forms of mental stimulation tend to have better memories than those who don't. Failure to stimulate cognitive function on a regular basis can actually lead to mental impairment.

314. LIMIT TIME SPENT WATCHING TELEVISION

The reasons behind a lack of mental stimulation are many. Some people become numbed by too much television, while others dull their brains with alcohol and other stupefying substances. Prescription and over-the-counter drug interactions can also impair cognitive function, as can certain medical conditions. But for the majority of older Americans, isolation and a lack of social interaction are the primary culprits. Social support means a lot of social interaction; we chat with friends, engage in a variety of activities, and live a relatively active life. All of this stimulates the brain on a number of important levels, keeping our cognitive skills well-honed. But older people who lack social support often have little to do to occupy their time except watch television. Opportunities to actually think, to exercise the brain, become increasingly limited. And with this lack of stimulation comes a subtle but serious reduction in mental functioning.

315. PUMP IT UP

As we age, we often experience difficulty understanding or completing math problems, and difficulty figuring out visual-spatial puzzles. While sometimes a sign of early dementia, these problems most often are simply the result of mental inactivity, of not sufficiently exercising the brain in these particular areas. Maintaining mental acuity is like training to be a professional athlete; you must pursue it full-time and with all the energy you have. The future results are too important for this to be a half-hearted venture. The key is training and practice. You must treat your brain like a muscle, giving it a workout on a regular basis.

316. TAKE MEMORIZATION CLASSES

Research has proved the success of training and practice when it comes to maintaining and strengthening our mental abilities. In one study, scientists evaluated the number of words people could recall after listening to a lengthy list of random words. Before they received memory training, the older members of the study group were able to recall fewer words than the younger members. But after just a handful of memory training sessions, which included tips such as placing words in meaningful groups rather than trying to memorize them out of context, the older participants were able to triple their word recall. In another study involving children, memorization training revealed an improvement in cognitive abilities not related to the memorization training and a leap in IQ test scores of 8 percent, as reported in the *Journal of the American Academy of Child and Adolescent Psychiatry.*

317. PAY ATTENTION

Many of us stumble through life only paying attention to what we absolutely have to and marginally noticing what we presume we can ignore. This may help us get by, but it does little for our brains and tricks us into missing a simple fact—being highly observant helps to sharpen our minds. Focusing intently on a particular project, new skill, or task hones your brain's ability to absorb information, order information, and retain information. Paying close attention, really focusing, essentially keeps your brain sharp and pliable.

318. RELIEVE STRESS AND DEPRESSION

Ronald Duman, professor of psychiatry and pharmacology at Yale University, has theorized that stress and depression not only kill brain cells, but also prevent new cells from being born. Stress produces glucocorticoids, which basically inform your brain that you are in danger. Your brain responds by maintaining a high state of alert, and if there is no resolution, those chemicals keep streaming through your blood, becoming, in effect, toxic to your brain. A brain on high alert is focused on survival, and thus has no time for rest and regeneration. Duman discovered that some antidepressants (Prozac in particular) and electroconvulsive therapy (shock treatments) seem to do more than relieve depression by boosting serotonin in the brain; they set off a neurochemical cascade that stimulate neurogenesis, or the production of new brain neurons. Duman theorizes that this neurogenesis may be what ultimately lifts someone out of depression. If you are living under very stressful conditions, do whatever you can to improve your situation. If you suffer from depression, seek medical help.

319. LOSE BELLY FAT

In a study of Kaiser Permanente patients in Northern California, middle-aged people with excess visceral fat—more commonly known as belly fat—were nearly three times more likely to suffer from dementia in their 70s and 80s than people with little to no belly fat. The researchers found these people have a much higher risk of having that visceral fat surrounding internal organs deep in their abdominal cavity. Doctors theorize that this fat may release toxins associated with atherosclerosis or the buildup of plaque in the brain that is frequently present in those afflicted with Alzheimer's. The study defined people who were 30 pounds or more overweight who had developed belly fat in their 40s were 3.6 times more likely to develop dementia. They reported that the risk for men with belly fat goes up when his waist exceeds 40 inches; for women, it's 35 inches. Doctors recommend a combination of weight training and aerobic exercise that targets the whole body (not just the abdominals), a low-fat diet, and minimal sugar. Surprisingly, recent research has suggested that including dairy products and getting plenty of sleep may help when it comes to battling belly fat.

320. GET PLENTY OF REST

Prolonged fatigue prevents the mind and body from functioning at optimal levels, depresses the immune system, and wears down the entire system—physical, mental, and emotional. Deep and genuine rest is transformative in many ways. Being in a state of true rest connects us to our intuitive levels and the innate pattern of health and well being residing within. Sleep allows the brain to juggle the input of new information to produce flashes of creative insight. It's fairly common to wake from a power nap with an "aha" moment. In other words, get plenty of rest—it's good for your brain! ✳

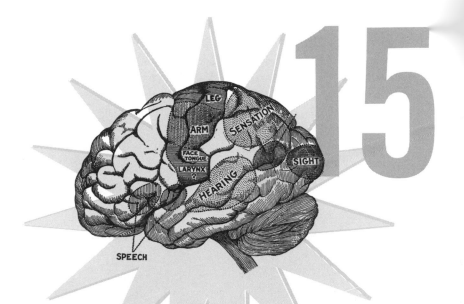

STIMULATE
YOUR
BRAIN

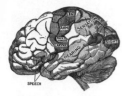

STIMULATE YOUR BRAIN

Arouse your passions for better brain health.

321. FREE YOUR MIND

Instead of worrying endlessly, take a walk, enjoy a shower, or do something repetitive, such as knitting or crocheting. Keeping part of your brain occupied with a repetitive action actually frees up the creative side of your brain to solve problems. This is why we often have great ideas when we are in the shower or not thinking about something in particular.

322. FALL IN LOVE

According to Dr. Frank Lawlis in *The IQ Answer*, falling in love stimulates your brain. "The act of loving someone can be directly observed through the brain and throughout your body. Your immune system sparkles with excitement that creates a better defense against disease, and you actually gain muscular strength. Your creativity soars from the stimulation of the right brain so even males begin to integrate their intellectual vision with creativity." He notes that the type of love doesn't matter as much as the depth of feeling. "We know that newborn babies thrive when loved, while those without love tend to suffer in mental strengths . . . evidence indicates that those who love the most gain the greatest benefit cognitively." Research has shown that falling in love raises levels of nerve growth for a sustained period of time, perhaps as much as a year. The hormones produced apparently help to restore the nervous system and trigger new growth.

323. DANCE, DANCE, DANCE

We all know that music and dance stimulate us in many ways. The rhythmic beats, melodies, and flowing physical movements all stimulate the senses and the brain. The areas most affected are the cerebellum, which has millions of nerve connections to the whole brain, including key connections to the frontal lobe; the motor ridge in the parietal lobe, which is considered the executive portion of brain activity; and the frontal regions. All are affected positively by rhythmic movements that involve balance and coordination. So choose songs that have moved you in the past or that elicited joyful, playful, or romantic feelings. Combine sexy music with a sensual dance, and you've not only relieved stress, you've limbered up—and juiced up—your brain and your body.

324. LISTEN TO MUSIC

Researchers have found that the same pleasure centers of the brain that are positively stimulated by food and sex are also affected by music. Any music that sends chills up your spine has a direct effect upon your mood. When we use music that is particularly stimulating to us in a positive way, we can elevate our mood, and feel more content, relaxed, energized, or turned on.

325. SING

Singing has been connected to intelligence, creativity, emotion, and memory, according to Daniel G. Amen, author of *Making a Good Brain Great*. It has been proven that singing information or attaching a melody or jingle to it helps you retain the information. "Singing stimulates temporal lobe function, an area of the brain heavily involved in memory," Dr. Amen reported. If you can't sing, try humming, which Dr. Amen said also provides a positive difference in mood and memory. "As the sound activates your brain, you will feel more alive and your brain will feel more tuned in to the moment."

326. FLIRT

According to Daniel G. Amen, MD, author of *Making a Good Brain Great*, when you feel an attraction to someone, areas deep in the brain, rich in the neurotransmitter dopamine, light up with pleasure. Extra dopamine courses through your body and brain, generating feelings of well-being. Your brain stem also activates, releasing phenylethylamine (PEA) which speeds the flow of information between nerve cells. "Taken together, the release of dopamine and PEA explains why, when we are around someone we feel attracted to, we feel a 'rush' and our hearts beat faster. Attraction is a powerful drug," reported Dr. Amen.

327. MAKE A COMMITMENT

When we choose a partner and commit to a mutually rewarding intimate relationship, we love on a deeper level, a more enduring level, and our brain produces the hormone oxytocin, known as "the bonding hormone." Women have higher levels of oxytocin, which may improve their ability to choose one partner (and also helps them bond with their newborns), while men's levels increase fivefold following orgasm. A Harvard University study found that married women are 20 percent less likely and married men 100 to 200 percent less likely to die of stress-related causes like heart disease, suicide, or cirrhosis of the liver than single people.

328. HAVE AN ORGASM

Orgasms are good on so many levels, obviously. Sex, in general, is stimulated by and stimulates the right hemisphere of your brain, the one associated with creativity, music, social skills, spirituality, and pleasure. During orgasm, blood flows into the right prefrontal cortex, creating that fabulous sense of release and gratification. Orgasms also stimulate deep emotional parts of the brain and thus provide a calming influence. Those who have orgasms experience less depression than those who do not. According to Werner Habermehl, a German sex researcher, the more sex you have, the smarter you become. He credits the stimulation of adrenaline and cortisol during lovemaking, plus the bonus surge of serotonin and endorphins that follows orgasm. Regular orgasms ultimately lead to a boost in self-esteem.

329. HAVE SEX REGULARLY

Sex not only feels good, it's good for you. Regular sexual activity is good for your brain, your mood, pain relief, and memory. Having an orgasm decreases pain activity by 50 percent. Having sex three times a week decreases heart attack and stroke by 50 percent. Regular sexual activity ultimately can help you live longer. This isn't just theory; it's clinical fact. A Duke University longitudinal study on aging found a strong correlation between the frequency and enjoyment of sexual intercourse and longevity. And a more recent British study had the same result, noting lower overall rates of mortality among men who have sex far more frequently than the once-a-week national average. Bottom line: Men and women who have frequent, loving sex tend to live longer than those who don't.

330. BAKE SOME BUNS

Researchers have found that certain foods with strong odors cause penile blood flow to increase. Dr. Alan R. Hirsch tested thirty scents and forty-six odors with men from ages eighteen to sixty-four. His results found that cinnamon buns caused the greatest arousal and that a combination of pumpkin pie and lavender caused an average increase in penile blood flow by 40 percent. Older men responded more to vanilla and men who had the best sex lives reported a preference for the aroma of strawberries. Every scent and odor that was used in the research caused some degree of increase in penile blood flow. Dr. Hirsch also studied the female reactions, which turned out to be markedly different. Among women between the ages of eighteen and forty, licorice was the most sexually stimulating. The combination of licorice and cucumber caused a 13 percent increase in vaginal blood flow. The pumpkin and lavender combination that the men liked so well caused an 11 percent increase. Women had negative responses to barbecue smoke, which caused a 14 percent decrease, and cherry, which caused an 18 percent decrease. In addition, they found that women had a 1 percent decrease in vaginal blood flow when they were exposed to a variety of men's colognes! So men—don't assume that your cologne is a turn-on for your woman.

331. EAT CHOCOLATE TO PERK YOU UP

Let's face it, chocolate lovers of America, one of the best things about chocolate is that "feel good lift" you get after eating a few pieces. It can be attributed to the caffeine present in small quantities or the theobromine, another weak stimulant, present in slightly higher amounts. However, the combination of these two, in tandem with the other 298 chemicals present, may just provide the "lift" that makes your day a little better. As a matter of fact, chocolate also contains phenylethylamine, a strong stimulant related to the amphetamine family, known to increase the activity of neurotransmitters in parts of the brain that control your ability to pay attention and stay alert.

332. TRY A SEXY HERB FROM PERU

The Peruvian herb maca, which has over 1000 years of safe use behind it, is proven to enhance libido and sexual function, according to Chris Kilham in *Better Nutrition* (September 1999). He says that maca, which is consumed throughout Peru, has achieved status as a bona fide aphrodisiac. Tests conducted on maca reveal no toxicity and a complete absence of adverse pharmacologic effects. Kilham writes: "For every health need, nature offers a solution, usually in the form of a safe, healthful plant. Maca may well provide tough competition for Viagra, and become a popular aphrodisiac—for men and women alike—in the United States." Search on Google for it and find out more . . . research is good for your brain.

333. TRY GINKGO BILOBA

We already noted that ginkgo biloba may be good for your brain, but there is evidence that it may also be good for your libido. Ginkgo has reportedly served as an aid to men who suffer from impotence induced by taking antidepressant medications. The recommended dosage is 120 to 240 milligrams daily, in 3 doses. Plan to take it for at least eight weeks before improvement shows. **Caution:** Ginkgo may interfere with antidepressant MAO-inhibitor drugs such as phenelzine sulfate (Nardil) or tranylcypromine (Parnate). If you're on heart medication and want to take ginkgo, consult your doctor first. And be sure to stick to the recommended dose of 120 to 240 milligrams a day.

334. TRY AN HERBAL TEA TO REVITALIZE YOUR LIBIDO

Sometimes depression or anxiety makes happy sexual functioning difficult. This may be because your energy is too low, or it may be connected with a hormone imbalance. Damiana stimulates both the nervous and hormonal systems, containing constituents that convert to hormones in the body. Vervain releases tension and stress and was traditionally used as an aphrodisiac. Wild oats and ginger are both stimulating, as well. Ginger is even said to fire the blood. Try the following recipe:

Energizing Tea

1 teaspoon dried damiana
1 teaspoon dried vervain
Put the herbs into a pot and add 2½ cups of boiling water. Steep for 10 minutes. Strain and flavor with licorice, ginger, or honey. Drink two cups a day. This will restore energy of all kinds, including sexual energy. ✴

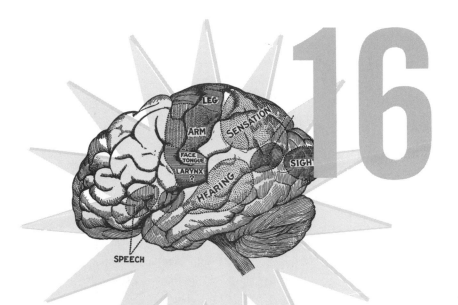

16

CHALLENGE
YOUR
BRAIN

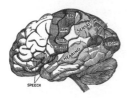

CHALLENGE YOUR BRAIN

Avoid the path of least resistance.

335. MAINTAIN MENTAL ACUITY

It's been said that we only use 10 percent of our brain. Keeping the brain strong and nimble isn't a quest just for seniors; it's something we should strive for throughout our lives. Exercise your brain regularly and vigorously, and you can virtually guarantee that cognitive function will remain in top form into your seventies, eighties, and beyond. Numerous studies have shown that people who lead lives with little mental stimulation experience greater cognitive loss as they age. Their memory fails with greater frequency, and they find it increasingly difficult to work puzzles, perform mathematic equations, and do other mental feats that come quite easily to people who "exercise" their brains often.

336. GET OFF THE COUCH

In a 2001 study published in the *Proceedings of the National Academy of Sciences*, some of the activities that led to less brain stimulation and increased risk of Alzheimer's included watching television, listening to music, attending social clubs, talking on the phone, visiting with friends, and attending religious services. These

188

were compared with reading books, studying a foreign language, and traveling. They found that any type of stimulating activity was more beneficial than none. The more intellectual the activity, however, the better it was for strengthening your brain muscles. It's a matter of engaging in life fully, having goals, having fun, and being interested in your surroundings, in other people, and in yourself. Sitting in front of the television set is not the best way to enjoy your life—or to challenge your brain.

337. PLAY THE NAME GAME

Enhance your memorization at every opportunity and take advantage of the challenges life presents every day. For example, at social events, or whenever introduced to someone new, repeat the person's name to yourself three times and then use it in conversation. Meet as many people as possible, and then test yourself the next morning to see how many you can remember. Give yourself bonus points for remembering how they were dressed or what they did for a living.

338. THROW AWAY THE GROCERY LIST

Another memory trick is to turn a grocery run into a game. After you've made a written list of your needs, memorize it to the best of your ability by taking a mental walk through your kitchen and pantry. Shop without referring to the list and see how well you've done before checking out. If your memory is sharp, you'll probably be able to remember almost everything. Since you shop for groceries often, this simple exercise will have a cumulative effect.

339. LEARN FIVE NEW WORDS A DAY

Like the athlete who takes time to warm up and flex his or her muscles before engaging in a strenuous activity, flexing your brain cells with a few basic word-play exercises warms up your mental engine. Words are fun; they expand your mind. Pick up your dictionary and pick out five words you don't know. Commit their definitions to memory and write five sentences using them in different ways. See if you can recite their definitions from memory the next day. And then learn five more. If you're not in the habit of using your mind to memorize poetry, song lyrics, obscure facts, or unfamiliar names, acquiring a new vocabulary can be a challenge. However, "practice makes perfect," and as you persevere, you'll soon discover that the task of committing words to memory will become increasingly easier to achieve and more satisfying.

340. LEARN TO PLAY A MUSICAL INSTRUMENT

According to Daniel G. Amen, author of *Making a Good Brain Great,* the College Entrance Examination Board in 1996 reported that students with experience in musical performance scored 51 points higher on the verbal part of the SAT and 39 points higher on the math section than the national average. "It [learning to play a musical instrument] teaches the brain new patterns and stimulates wide areas of the cortex. . . . Learning a musical instrument, at any age, can be helpful in developing and activating temporal lobe neurons. As the temporal lobes are activated in an effective way, they are more likely to have improved function overall," Dr. Amen said. In another study, music majors were the most likely group of college grads to be admitted to medical school (66 percent, the highest percentage of any group).

341. PRACTICE NEW SKILLS

Learning, as you may recall from your school days, involves understanding and memorization. As you become familiar with novel ideas, newly presented information, or a new vocabulary, your brain becomes much more receptive to retaining further knowledge if you take the time to review and practice what you have already learned. It's a good idea, therefore, to open your notebook and review the previously studied vocabulary before you turn to the next set of words. Your brain, like the rest of your body, is capable of achieving new skills.

342. AVOID CLICHÉS

Cliché is the French word for "stereotype." In other words, it's something that is worn-out through repetitive use. In English, *cliché* is used to describe phrases and expressions that have crept into the language to such an extent that they have lost their freshness and original meaning. Clichés are boring and trite, yet we continue to parrot them, scarcely aware of how they clutter our speech. "Saved by the bell" is an example of a cliché. Relying on cliché is lazy. Exercise your brain by challenging yourself to avoid clichés and come up with a fresh metaphor or an original expression. And maybe you'll create a new cliché that lazy people can use when they talk.

343. REPLACE PROFANITY WITH A SHARPENED VOCABULARY

It is deplorable and disheartening how obscenity has infiltrated our lives and language. Characters in books, actors in movies, rappers, men, women, and children shamelessly rattle off strings of ugly obscenities without thought or pause. There was a time when mothers washed their kids' mouths with soap for saying a disreputable word. Now mothers use words that would make a sailor blush. Nevertheless, there is still a segment of society that will not tolerate profanity. Persons wishing to advance professionally in a chosen career should guard against slips of the tongue. Rather than flinging profane words in the heat of an argument, make it your goal to broaden your vocabulary and to use words that really express how you feel. Tax your brain by challenging it to learn and remember a lexicon that will express your frustration gracefully.

344. MOVE BEYOND SLANG

Slang is not necessarily a lexicon of obscene words. Depending on which stratum of society is speaking, some of the vocabulary may be offensive. Slang originated as the secret speech of tramps and thieves and other unsavory characters. Urban street gangs probably belong in that category. Basically, slang that is not offensive is Teen Speak, and its main characteristic is that the words are short-lived. But relying on slang to express yourself is another sign of a lazy brain. A mind focused on slang is creative in the way it invents or assigns a new meaning to a common word; but a clever mind challenges itself to learn new words that more appropriately and fully express its thoughts. Or be really clever and create your own slang.

345. STUDY LATIN

As we know, at the height of its glory, the Roman Empire was an octopus reaching out its imperial tentacles north and south, east and west, invading and occupying territories. Wherever they went, the Romans left imprints of their language and culture. Inevitably, the Latin spoken by Roman troops influenced European languages. Latin remains a powerful force—the law and the sciences still retain their specialized Latin lexicons. Latin formed the basis for French, Spanish, and Italian. Studying Latin will challenge your brain, help build your vocabulary, and help you learn to read or speak other languages.

346. PLAY TRIVIA GAMES

Trivia games can be marvelous ways to see how good you are at jogging your memory. When you're digging around in those dusty corners of your mind to dig up the answer, your brain synapses will be firing, ruffling through your mental files. It's even fair to buy a game, read all the answer cards and then test how well you are at remembering something freshly learned. Read the cards often and play against yourself to see how much you improve.

347. PLAY GAMES

According to Dr. Frank Lawlis in *The IQ Answer*, an idle brain loses brainpower: "It [your brain] begins to lose the dendrite connections with major centers, and receptor sites fall away, blocking the passage of neuron transmissions. . . . Just as physical exercise generates strength in various parts of the body, mental exercise builds strength in various parts of the brain. Individual mental exercises generally affect the three areas of the front (executive region), temporal (memory), and occipital lobes (visual imagery)." Lawlis recommends bridge, chess, poker, bingo, and charades. He also recommends games favored by Mensa (an organization of brainiacs, those who rank in the top 2 percent when it comes to IQ), such as Brainstrain, Cityscape, Cube Checkers, Doubles Wild, Finish Lines, and many more that can be found in the American Mensa Library.

348. WORK PUZZLES

Stimulate your brain by doing puzzles, such as the daily crossword puzzle, anagrams, find-a-word, and maze games. Puzzles are a great way to strengthen and maintain several different areas of cognitive function, including memory and visual-spatial areas. Puzzle books can be purchased very inexpensively and are a great way to kill time while waiting in line or for an appointment. Instead of buying celebrity or puff magazines, buy puzzle magazines. Crosswords, word-search puzzles, Sudoku, and other puzzles are all good ways to occupy your mind without stressing it. These activities will keep your brain fit, too. Just try to find puzzles that match your skill level. Puzzles that are too difficult will add stress, not reduce it!

349. READ THE CLASSICS

Read as much as you can and focus on works that challenge you. The latest pot-boiler may be a fun read, but it's probably as mentally challenging as a Dick and Jane primer. You can give your brain a workout by reading a literary classic you've always meant to tackle or by reading a nonfiction book on a topic you're interested in but know nothing about. Read carefully, with memory and recall in mind. To help you assimilate this new information, discuss it with friends.

350. JOIN A BOOK CLUB

This has a triple bonus. Most book clubs pick challenging books and set a specific deadline for reading them. Part of the fun is analyzing a book's structure, theme, characterizations, plot, and other concepts that may not be familiar to you, but that will be a lot of fun, as well as mentally challenging. Also, groups typically gather for discussions, offering you opportunities to socialize, engage in meaningful conversation, and invigorate yourself. It's also likely to help you stay contemporary, and keep up with what's going on in the world. Join a book club; it's a win-win-win situation.

351. TAKE A CLASS

Education is never a bad thing, and studies have shown that the more education you receive, the better your mental acuity—and the longer you will retain it. Take a class that challenges your thought processes, rather than something with which you're already familiar. Most community colleges and universities offer continuing education classes on a wide variety of subjects, and many sessions are held at night to accommodate people who work during the day. And choose a challenging subject, something that forces you to think or flexes brain cells you haven't used for eons.

352. TEACH A CLASS

Teach a continuing education class. In addition to the joy that comes with sharing your life wisdom, teaching helps strengthen mental function through reading, self-learning, and lecturing. Everyone is adept at something, so choose your specialty, approach a local continuing education program, and improve the world with your knowledge. You don't need a teaching degree, just experience.

353. STUDY THE HUMAN BODY

You are the one who is responsible for the upkeep of your body. It's the only one you have. Your body is an extremely complex, finely tuned, and yet remarkably efficient machine. Many of us take better care of our cars than we do our bodies. When something goes wrong with our automobile, we immediately take it to a mechanic. Most of us know exactly what the mechanic is talking about when he or she tells us that this part of the car needs replacement or adjustment. The question is how well do we know the physiological makeup of our bodies? When a physician uses a scientific term in reference to a possible ailment, is the word familiar? Studying human physiology will challenge your brain (memorize the official names for your collarbone or your leg bones and what your pituitary gland does), improve your ability to visualize what's going on in your body, and help you understand the complex terminology doctors will use when discussing your health.

354. LEARN A FOREIGN LANGUAGE

Being multilingual is extremely beneficial these days, and learning a foreign language can also be quite mentally challenging because it requires the thoughtful assimilation of new information and a strong memory. Struggle with those verbs, pore over grammatical structure, force yourself to speak it at every opportunity, and stick with it even when it seems futile. The minute it feels like your brain is stretching, you're already succeeding. Once you've learned a new language, reward yourself with a vacation to the country that speaks it so that you can practice speaking the new language and learn more about its culture.

355. FIND A NEW HOBBY

According to Daniel G. Amen, MD, in *Making a Good Brain Great*, it's far better to learn something new than to repeat the same activities: "The best mental exercise is acquiring new knowledge and doing things that you haven't done before . . . when the brain does something over and over, even a complicated task, it learns how to do it using less and less energy." Find a hobby that requires coordination between multiple brain regions, such as ballroom dancing, painting, or learning a musical instrument. Knitting, photography, woodworking, gardening, writing poetry, or anything that requires you to study something new will also stimulate your brain. Don't take the easy way out either; pick something that challenges you and then strive to do it well. All of these activities will strengthen and maintain mental acuity on a variety of levels.

356. IMPROVE YOUR MATH SKILLS

Improve your mathematic abilities by doing calculations in your head whenever possible. For example, balance your checkbook without the aid of a calculator, and mentally figure out sales tax and how much change you should get back whenever you make a purchase. Reliance on technology tends to dull our math skills, a situation that only worsens with age. Buy some of the myriad of math puzzle books and give them a whirl. If you really want to challenge your brain, study advanced mathematics or chemistry.

357. WRITE YOUR AUTOBIOGRAPHY

This can be a very rewarding activity in that you preserve your life experiences for the benefit of other family members and exercise your brain in the process. Recalling previous events requires a strong memory (which may be aided by going through photo albums, letters, etc.), and the act of writing improves visual-spatial skills. If you've lived a truly extraordinary life, consider getting your memoirs published.

358. KEEP A JOURNAL

Keeping a daily journal will inspire you to think about your life, patterns in your life, what you're really thinking, etc. Formulating thoughts and writing them down will benefit your brain in multiple ways, particularly if you strive for complexity, expand your vocabulary, or become more observant. It will also help relieve stress, particularly if you dispel your worries onto the page and truly release them.

359. WRITE POETRY

It doesn't matter if you are really bad at writing poetry. That's precisely the reason to do it. Poetry is a creative form of writing that is indeed a fine art. Try your hand at various styles, such as:

► An epic poem that celebrates, in a grand style, mythological and actual historical events
► An ode that is a lyric poem (An ode is a lyrical dedication to something or someone that the writer admires and loves. It describes how the subject of the ode affects the poet emotionally.)
► A narrative poem that tells a story in a somewhat simpler style. "Paul Revere's Ride" by the American poet Henry Wadsworth Longfellow is a narrative poem.

Lyric poems are sensitive in tone. They express the poet's personal feelings of love, yearning, sorrow, and happiness. Poetry can rhyme or not; poems that do not rhyme are referred to as blank verse. A great deal of poetry has a definite repetitive rhythm. Writing poetry will help you get in touch with your feelings, help you think metaphorically, and (unless you are an accomplished poet) tax your brain.

360. TURN EVERYTHING INTO A LEARNING EVENT

If you are planning a trip to a museum, study the progression of art, learning the artists and the era, such as Byzantine, Cubism, Impressionism, Renaissance, etc. See how much you can memorize and then use your knowledge to impress your companion. You can also do this for stargazing, classical music concerts, opera, theater, etc. You can even do this when going to a basketball game or skiing. Not only will you stimulate your brain, you'll impress your friends.

361. WATCH PBS

PBS offers intelligent programming that will inform, educate, and stimulate your brain. Forgo the mindless and mind-numbing shows that commercial stations use to fill the airwaves. In the same way we become what we think (or eat), we also become what we watch. Do you seriously want to clutter your brain with the equivalent of junk food? Pick and choose carefully, and choose shows that stimulate or educate your brain. It will not only make you mentally sharp, it will liven up your conversation when socializing.

362. JOG YOUR MEMORY

Memory is made and reinforced by the strength of connections between nerve cells and the formation of memory-storage protein molecules inside nerve cells. When a memory of a new idea is formed, like a name or an address, thousands of nerve cells are involved. If you don't use that bit of memory shortly after, it will soon fade away. But if you use it and reactivate the memory many times, you reinforce the stored chemical protein molecules that make up that memory. Reading these words creates thousands of electrochemical reactions in your brain. Often the brain is referred to as a computer, but the malleability and interactivity of the brain is far beyond any computer that is presently in use or on the horizon. One way to challenge your brain is to work on improving your memory. Try memorizing lines of your favorite poems and see if you can recite them for the next seven days. Your electrochemicals will love you for it.

363. RECONSIDER RETIREMENT

We must exercise the brain as if it were a muscle. We have all heard the stories of the dangers of retiring and not having a plan of how to fill your time. The stories are true, and the science is there to prove it. Most aspects of work, even the commute, the interaction with others, and the daily challenges, are stimulating. When you retire, if you don't build in challenges for your brain and body, then you can suffer physical decline and even mental decline. Studies also find that the more intellectually stimulating the job, the less likely Alzheimer's will strike.

364. USE IT OR LOSE IT

A 1993 experiment with two groups of mice showed the importance of exercising the brain. The first group was placed in a barren cage with no mental stimulation. They just ate, slept, or wandered around their cage. The second group was trained in running complex mazes.

After a few weeks, an electron microscope was used to compare the nerve cells of the trained mice to those of the untrained group. There was a noticeable difference between the two groups. The maze mice had developed wider and longer nerve dendrites and more synapses than the couch-potato mice. In the next phase of the study, the maze group was put in solitary confinement without stimulation. At the end of several more weeks, their brains were examined. They no longer had enhanced dendrites and synapses; they had all shrunken away, and their brains were as if they had never been trained. "Use it or lose it" was the conclusion of this study. In another study, it took only four days for dendrites and synapses to flare out and grow when toys were put in cages along with laboratory animals.

365. BE CREATIVE

Creativity goes beyond thinking, beyond the gathering and assimilation of information. Creativity is what happens in your brain when you relax and allow your brain to birth new thoughts, new ways of seeing, or new ways of doing. According to Dr. Frank Lawlis, author of *The IQ Answer*, when we focus on problems, we use our brains to establish "rational relationships and cogent associations." Dr. Lawlis says a problem-solving brain emits Lobeta waves indicative of the process of transferring information from one area of the brain to another. When you enter a creative state, however, Dr. Lawlis believes your brain enters the Theta state in which your frontal lobe shuts down, allowing other lobes to light up. In this creative state, the occipital lobe (imagery) and the temporal lobe (memory) activate. In effect, your brain goes into a sort of blissful, hypnotic state that often results in creative works of art. Achieving a creative state of mind can be almost as restorative as deep sleep. So challenge your brain by releasing it to work its magic. ✳